FIBROMYALGIA

Thanthullu Vasu

tfm Publishing Limited, Castle Hill Barns, Harley, Shrewsbury, SY5 6LX, UK
Tel: +44 (0)1952 510061; Fax: +44 (0)1952 510192
E-mail: info@tfmpublishing.com; Web site: www.tfmpublishing.com

Editing: Dr. Christine Graham PhD
Editing, design & typesetting: Nikki Bramhill BSc (Hons), Dip Law
Cover photo: © iStock.com
Dotted silhouette of person
Credit: StudioM1; stock illustration ID: 920258130

First edition:	© 2022
Paperback	ISBN: 978-1-913755-24-9
E-book editions:	© 2022
Epub	ISBN: 978-1-913755-25-6
Mobi	ISBN: 978-1-913755-26-3
Web pdf	ISBN: 978-1-913755-27-0

Printed by Gutenberg Press Ltd., Gudja Road, Tarxien, GXQ 2902, Malta
Tel: +356 2398 2201; Fax: +356 2398 2290
E-mail: info@gutenberg.com.mt; Web site: www.gutenberg.com.mt

Contents

Section 3: Clinical examination

Section 4: Education

Section 5: Physical therapies

Section 6: Complementary therapies

Section 7: Medications

Section 8: Injection therapies

Section 9: Psychological therapies

Preface

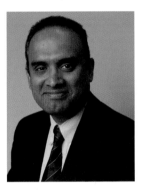

To live is to suffer, to survive is to find some meaning in the suffering.

Friedrich Nietzsche/Gordon Allport

Fibromyalgia causes widespread pain all over the body with significant fatigue; it can affect cognitive performance, physical skills, psychological status, ability to work, and social life, and can debilitate the affected patient. Patients with fibromyalgia syndrome experience unrefreshing sleep and brain fog. Scientific evidence has clearly shown that these individuals have a poor quality of life. Fibromyalgia affects not only the individual patients but also their family and social contacts. Their self-identity is also affected because of the condition.

Fibromyalgia can affect 2% of the population; many go through a 'revolving door' phenomenon of seeing many specialists and professionals before diagnosis. This journey can take as long as a few years and causes significant frustration among patients, losing confidence in the healthcare system. This book was written to increase awareness and knowledge in healthcare professionals when seeing these patients in their practice and to empower patients with the ability to take control of the condition into their own hands.

Fibromyalgia presents with a wide spectrum of symptoms and accompanying comorbidities. In addition, many functional pain syndromes can co-exist with fibromyalgia. The disease is associated with a huge financial burden and causes a significant economic impact in all countries; in the USA, it is estimated that fibromyalgia accounts for the loss of 1–2% of the country's overall productivity.

> *Plus ça change, plus c'est la même chose.*
> *[The more things change, the more they remain the same.]*
> **Jean-Baptiste Alphonse Karr**

In a survey among doctors in Scandinavia, fibromyalgia was rated as the 'least prestigious' disease. If this is the situation among healthcare professionals, it could be worse among the lay public, who have no medical knowledge of the condition and its disastrous effects on various body systems.

Patients with fibromyalgia often feel that they are not believed and are not listened to. Despite knowledge and an evidence base on this disease and the definitive diagnostic criteria and management pathways, healthcare systems fail the affected suffering patients in many parts of the world.

> *Chronic pain might be unavoidable, but suffering is optional!*

As fibromyalgia affects patients physically, emotionally, and socially, a biopsychosocial model to look at self-management strategies is the best approach and is backed by proper scientific evidence. Furthermore, a holistic approach looking at multimodal therapies with rehabilitation programmes with individual need assessments helps in a better recovery pathway. This book gives a detailed description of the various aspects of fibromyalgia syndrome. It will motivate patients to engage in a self-management pathway, giving them the confidence and skills to take control into their own hands.

Out of suffering have emerged the strongest souls;
the most massive characters are seared with scars.

Khalil Gibran

I have tried to keep this book simple and clear, but at the same time, based on available scientific evidence. I do not believe in a single miracle cure or a magic wand to erase fibromyalgia. It's important that patients are thoroughly informed to equip them with the skills and confidence required to take control of the condition into their own hands. The book will also help healthcare professionals to understand this suffering, show empathy and kindness, and make the world a better place to live for these frustrated patients.

I thank Nikki Bramhill from tfm Publishing, who strongly encouraged my idea for this fibromyalgia book and supported me throughout the journey with passion and motivation. This book is my fourth published by tfm Publishing, and I am amazed by their team's constant enthusiasm and support. I also thank Christine Graham, Science and Medical Editor (STEM) and indexer, who has done a marvellous job editing the book in such an elegant, swift way. Without both their help, this book could not have been possible.

To all the readers, I thank you very much for reading this book. All your feedback is much appreciated. If this book helps to raise the profile of fibromyalgia thus creating more awareness, lobby the need for services for patients suffering from fibromyalgia and empower patients with more skills to cope, then the aim of this book will have been achieved. This book is dedicated to all clinicians who have listened empathetically to the suffering of patients affected with fibromyalgia.

Dr Thanthullu Vasu MBBS MD DNB FRCA FFPMRCA Dip Pain Mgt
Consultant in Pain Medicine
University Hospitals of Leicester NHS Trust, UK

Abreviations

5-HT	5-hydroxytryptamine
ABCT	Attachment-based compassion therapy
ACR	American College of Rheumatology
ACT	Acceptance and commitment therapy
ACTH	Adrenocorticotrophic hormone
ACTTION	Analgesic, Anaesthetic, and Addiction Clinical Trial Translations Innovations Opportunities and Networks
APS	American Pain Society
APT	Adaptive pacing therapy
ASIC	Acid-sensing ion channel
ATP	Adenosine triphosphate
AVS	Arteriole-venule shunt
AWMF	Arbeitsgemeinschaft der Wissenschaftlichen Medizinischen Fachgesellschaften e.V. (Association of the Scientific Medical Societies in Germany)
BDNF	Brain-derived neurotrophic factor
BoNT-A	Botulinum toxin type A
BoNT-B	Botulinum toxin type B
BPI	Brief Pain Inventory
BPS	British Pain Society
cAMP	Cyclic adenosine monophosphate
CBD	Cannabidiol
CBN	Cannabinol
CBT	Cognitive behavioural therapy
CBT-i	Cognitive behavioural therapy for insomnia
CBT-p	Cognitive behavioural therapy for pain
CFS	Chronic fatigue syndrome

CGRP	Calcitonin gene-related peptide
COMT	Catechol-O-methyltransferase
COX	Cyclo-oxygenase
COX-1	Cyclo-oxygenase-1
COX-2	Cyclo-oxygenase-2
CPAQ	Chronic Pain Acceptance Questionnaire
CPCI	Chronic Pain Coping Inventory
CPET	Cardiopulmonary exercise testing
CRF-LI	Corticotropin-releasing factor-like immunoreactivity
CRH	Corticotrophin-releasing hormone
CRP	C-reactive protein
CSF	Cerebrospinal fluid
DHEA	Dehydroepiandrosterone
DOP	Delta (δ) opioid
DPA	Data Protection Act
DSM-IV	Diagnostic and Statistical Manual for Mental Disorders
ECG	Electrocardiogram
EEG	Electroencephalography
EMDR	Eye movement desensitisation and reprocessing
EMG	Electromyography
EQ-5D	EuroQol 5D score
ESR	Erythrocyte sedimentation rate
EULAR	European League Against Rheumatism (more recently, European Alliance of Associations for Rheumatology)
FDA	Food and Drug Administration
FIQ	Fibromyalgia Impact Questionnaire
FMA UK	Fibromyalgia Action UK
fMRI	Functional magnetic resonance imaging
FPM	Faculty of Pain Medicine
GABA	Gamma-aminobutyric acid
GET	Graded exercise therapy
GH	Growth hormone
GHB	Gamma-hydroxybutyrate
GluN	Glutamate

GMP	Good Medical Practice
GnRH	Gonadotropin-releasing hormone
HADS	Hospital Anxiety and Depression Scale
HCPC	Health & Care Professions Council
HIV	Human immunodeficiency virus
HPA axis	Hypothalamic-pituitary-adrenal axis
HPG axis	Hypothalamic-pituitary-gonadal axis
HRQoL	Health-related quality of life
HRV	Heart rate variability
IAPT	Improving Access to Psychological Therapies
IASP	International Association for the Study of Pain
ICD	International Classification of Disease
IGF-I	Insulin-like growth factor I
IL-1β	Interleukin-1 beta
IMPROvE	Interdisciplinary Rehabilitation and Evaluation Programme for Patients With Chronic Widespread Pain: Randomized Controlled Trial
iNOS	Inducible nitric oxide synthase
JNK	c-Jun N-terminal kinase
KOP	Kappa (κ) opioid
LT	Leukotriene
MAOI	Monoamine oxidase inhibitor
MBCT	Mindfulness-based cognitive therapy
MBSR	Mindfulness-based stress reduction
ME	Myalgic encephalomyelitis
MET	Metabolic equivalent of task
MOP	Mu (μ) opioid
MOR	μ-opioid receptor
MRI	Magnetic resonance imaging
NAPQI	N-acetyl-p-benzoquinone imine
NASEM	National Academies of Sciences, Engineering, and Medicine
NFA	National Fibromyalgia Association
NFMCPA	National Fibromyalgia & Chronic Pain Association
NGF	Nerve growth factor
NHS	National Health Service

NICE	National Institute for Health and Care Excellence
NMDA	N-methyl-D-aspartate
NNH	Number needed to harm
NNT	Number needed to treat
N/OFQ	Nociceptin/orphanin FQ
NREM	Non-rapid eye movement
NRLS	National Reporting and Learning System
NSAID	Non-steroidal anti-inflammatory drug
P	Phosphorus
PACE	Pacing, graded Activity, and Cognitive behaviour therapy; a randomised Evaluation trial
PASS	Pain Anxiety Symptoms Scale
PCS	Pain Catastrophising Scale
PET	Positron emission tomography
PG	Prostaglandin
PGE1	Prostaglandin E1
PGE2	Prostaglandin E2
PGI2	Prostaglandin I2
PGIC	Patients' Global Impression of Change
PMP	Pain management programme
PRF	Pulsed radiofrequency
PTSD	Post-traumatic stress disorder
QALY	Quality-adjusted life-year
QoL	Quality of life
rCBF	Regional cerebral blood flow
RCT	Randomised controlled trial
REM	Rapid eye movement
RFC	Residual functional capacity
rs-fMRI	Resting-state functional magnetic resonance imaging
SF	Short-Form
SIGN	Scottish Intercollegiate Guidelines Network
SNAP-25	Synaptosomal-associated protein 25
SNARE	Soluble N-ethylmaleimide-sensitive factor attachment protein receptor
SNRI	Serotonin-noradrenaline reuptake inhibitor

SOCRATES	Site, onset, characteristics, radiation, associations, timing, exacerbating/relieving factors, severity
SOPA	Survey of Pain Attitudes
SPECT	Single-photon emission computed tomography
SS	Symptom Severity
SSRI	Selective serotonin reuptake inhibitor
TACE	Tumour necrosis factor alpha-converting enzyme
TENS	Transcutaneous electrical nerve stimulation
THC	Tetrahydrocannabinol
TNF	Tumour necrosis factor
TRPV-1	Transient receptor potential vanilloid 1
TRPV-2	Transient receptor potential vanilloid 2
TXA2	Thromboxane A2
VAS	Visual analogue score
VO_2	Volume of oxygen consumption
WHO	World Health Organization
WPI	Widespread Pain Index

Section 1

Introduction

Fibromyalgia

Chapter 1

History of fibromyalgia

Introduction

The term 'fibromyalgia' was coined in 1976 by P. K. Hench. It comes from the Latin word *fibro* meaning fibrotic tissue, and from the Greek word *myo* meaning muscle and *algos* meaning pain. Initially, fibromyalgia was mistakenly thought to be a psychiatric disorder. However, it was only in the 19th century that it was described as a rheumatological disorder associated with stiffness, pain, fatigue and difficulty with sleeping.

History before the 20th century

In 1592, the French physician Guillaume de Baillou introduced the term 'muscular rheumatism' to denote musculoskeletal pain that did not originate from injury.

In 1815, the Scottish surgeon William Balfour was the first person to describe 'tender points' which are painful areas on application of pressure (see Chapter 14 for details). At around that time, many clinicians believed the symptoms of fibromyalgia resulted from inflammation and in 1904, the term 'fibrositis' was used by W. R. Gowers. In the same year, R. Stockman described painful nodules and hyperplasia in inflammatory connective tissue. Various other terms were also used by other scientists, including psychogenic rheumatism, muscular fibrositis, neurasthaenia, myelasthaenia and non-articular rheumatism.

History from the late 20th century

In 1947, E. W. Boland was the first person to recognise the functional aspect of fibromyalgia, rather than focusing purely on the physical findings, and used the term 'psychogenic rheumatism'. In 1968, Eugene Traut published that there is a female preponderance of the condition, along with an association with headaches.

In 1977, Smythe and Moldofsky described the clinical characteristics of fibromyalgia, detailing widespread pain and tenderness noted in this condition. They recognised that the tender points are more sensitive on palpation in patients with this condition, compared with healthy controls. They also described various other associated characteristics, including sleep problems, tiredness and emotional involvement. They identified non-refreshing sleep and tender points with pain as two key features of fibromyalgia.

In 1981, Yunus used the term 'fibromyalgia' in scientific publications when describing this condition. He was the first to propose a formal set of three categories of criteria to diagnose fibromyalgia: (1) obligatory, (2) major and (3) minor.

In the 1980s, conditions including irritable bowel, bladder problems and migraine were first described as being associated with fibromyalgia. At the same time, formal diagnostic criteria for fibromyalgia began to emerge in the literature.

Fibromyalgia formally recognised as a disease

The American Medical Association recognised fibromyalgia syndrome as a disease in 1987. The first formal diagnostic criteria for fibromyalgia using tender points were proposed by the American College of Rheumatology and published in 1990. The presence of 11 of a total of 18 tender points was required for diagnosis. These diagnostic criteria enabled research to focus on various aspects of the disease, and were widely accepted by the medical community (see Chapter 14 for details).

In 1991, the Fibromyalgia Impact Questionnaire (FIQ) was developed to evaluate the functional outcome of fibromyalgia. In 2005, the American Pain Society published its first guidelines for management of the condition.

In 2007, the United States Food and Drug Administration (FDA) approved the first drug for the treatment of fibromyalgia, namely pregabalin (brand name Lyrica®). It should be noted that pregabalin was commonly prescribed and used off-licence prior to its FDA approval.

Widespread Pain Index instead of trigger points

In 2010, the Widespread Pain Index (WPI), which assesses symptom severity, among a number of criteria, was developed as a diagnostic tool for fibromyalgia, thereby replacing the traditional use of tender points as the basis for diagnosis of the condition (see Chapter 14 for detailed discussion). This novel system thus helps to rule out observer bias when making the diagnosis. More recently, in 2016, new criteria have been proposed by the American College of Rheumatology, based on bedside clinical measures of central sensitisation such as evoked pain responses.

Famous people who have suffered from fibromyalgia

It is thought that famous historic figures including Charles Darwin (1809–1882) and artist Frida Kahlo (1907–1954) might have suffered from fibromyalgia. Interestingly, the 12th May is annually commemorated as the International Fibromyalgia Awareness Day, in honour of the birthday of Florence Nightingale (1820–1910) who also suffered from the condition.

Current celebrities reported in the media with fibromyalgia include American singer-songwriter Lady Gaga, film actor Morgan Freeman, Grammy Award winning singer and songwriter Sinead O'Connor, comedian Janeane Garofalo, British model Jo Guest and singer Rosie Hamlin.

History of patient groups

Fibromyalgia Action UK is a registered charity that was set up in 1992 to provide support to people with fibromyalgia. It is almost entirely run by volunteers. To date, there are many fibromyalgia patient support groups and forums, which are discussed in more detail in Chapter 66.

Key Points

- Various terms were used over the last five centuries to describe fibromyalgia symptoms.
- The term 'fibromyalgia' was coined by P. K. Hench in 1976.
- Other conditions associated with fibromyalgia were first described in the 1970s and 1980s.
- In 1990, the American College of Rheumatology proposed formal criteria to enable a standardised diagnostic process for fibromyalgia, as well as for research purposes.
- These diagnostic criteria were updated in 2010, with the Widespread Pain Index, including symptom severity scores, replacing the trigger point method traditionally used for diagnosis.

References

1. Baillou G. *Liber de rheumatismo et pleuritide dorsali.* Paris: Thevart MJ; 1642.

2. Gowers WR. The development of the concept of fibrositis. *Br Med J* 1904; 1(2246): 17-21.

3. Boland EW. Psychogenic rheumatism: the musculoskeletal expression of psychoneurosis. *Ann Rheum Dis* 1947; 6(4): 195-203.

4. Stockman R. The causes, pathology, and treatment of chronic rheumatism. *Edinb Med J* 1904; 15: 107-16.

5.   Hench PK. Nonarticular rheumatism, 22nd rheumatism review: review of the American and English literature for the years 1973 and 1974. *Arthritis Rheum* 1976; 19: 1081-9.

6.   Higuera V. Fibromyalgia: real or imagined?; 2020. Available from: https://www.healthline.com/health/fibromyalgia-real-or-imagined.

7.   Smythe HA, Moldofsky H. Two contributions to understanding of the 'fibrositis' syndrome. *Bull Rheum Dis* 1977-1978; 28(1): 928-31.

8.   Yunus M, Masi AT, Calabro JJ, *et al*. Primary fibromyalgia (fibrositis): clinical study of 50 patients with matched normal controls. *Semin Arthritis Rheum* 1981; 11(1): 151-71.

9.   Inanici F, Yunus MB. History of fibromyalgia: past to present. *Curr Pain Headache Rep* 2004; 8(5): 369-78.

10.   Wolfe F, Smythe HA, Yunus MB, *et al*. The American College of Rheumatology 1990 criteria for the classification of fibromyalgia. Report of the multicenter Criteria Committee. *Arthritis Rheum* 1990; 33(2): 160-72.

11.   Wolfe F. The clinical syndrome of fibrositis. *Am J Med* 1986; 81(3A): 7-14.

12.   Wolfe F, Clauw DJ, Fitzcharles MA, *et al*. The American College of Rheumatology preliminary diagnostic criteria for fibromyalgia and measurement of symptom severity. *Arthritis Care Res* 2010; 62(5): 600-10.

13.   Fibromyalgia Action UK; 2020. The history of fibromyalgia. Available from: https://www.fmauk.org/latest-news-mainmenu-2/articles-1/1388-the-history-of-fibromyalgia.

14.   Cherney K. 5 celebrities with fibromyalgia; 2017. Available from: https://www.healthline.com/health/celebrities-fibromyalgia.

Chapter 2

What is fibromyalgia?

Introduction

This chapter will provide a brief introduction on fibromyalgia. Clinical features of the condition and its diagnostic criteria will be elaborated in Chapters 13 and 14, respectively. Different aspects of fibromyalgia will also be discussed in detail in later chapters.

Functional pain syndromes

The International Association for the Study of Pain (IASP) describes functional pain syndromes as conditions in which patients complain of physical pain or discomfort, with no physiological or organic cause identified despite extensive diagnostic testing. According to the IASP, functional pain syndromes comprise a spectrum of conditions (see Chapter 13), including:

- Somatic conditions:
  - fibromyalgia;
  - low back pain;
  - temporomandibular joint disorders;
  - vulvodynia.
- Visceral conditions:
  - irritable bowel syndrome;
  - painful bladder syndrome;
  - sensitive heart.

- Comorbid conditions:
  - chronic fatigue syndrome.

In the majority of fibromyalgia sufferers, many of the above conditions may coexist.

Presentation of fibromyalgia

Fibromyalgia is a chronic idiopathic condition and is characterised by widespread pain in various areas of the body, and associated with symptoms including fatigue, waking up feeling unrefreshed and impaired cognitive function. Other associations have been described, including sleep impairment, emotional distress and memory and concentration difficulties (also called 'fibro-fog' or 'brain fog'). Details on how to make a diagnosis of fibromyalgia, including the use of diagnostic scoring, are explained in Chapter 14.

Prevalence

Approximately 2–8% of the general population are affected by fibromyalgia. According to published reports, approximately 1.76 million adults in England and Wales, and 4 million adults (2% of the population) in the USA have this condition.

Fibromyalgia is at least twice as common in women as in men, with a study in a general population reporting a prevalence of 3.4% in females and only 0.5% in men.

Fibromyalgia can affect individuals in any age groups, including children. Of note, women are particularly affected between the ages of 30 and 60 years.

Another study showed a higher prevalence of fibromyalgia in urban areas (0.7–11.4%), compared with rural areas (0.1–5.2%). Furthermore, the prevalence of fibromyalgia was found to be significantly lower in developing countries than in developed countries.

A meta-analysis of nine studies reported a prevalence of 2–4% in adults and 6.2% in children, showing that the condition is also common in children.

Fibromyalgia is commonly associated with comorbidities. A study published in 2015 showed that 73% of patients with fibromyalgia had another diagnosis, in addition to fibromyalgia.

A recent meta-analysis of 23 studies showed a median incidence of chronic widespread pain of 12.5 per 1000 person-years, which increased to 67 per 1000 person-years in patients with pre-existing pain. The same meta-analysis also described a median incidence of physician-diagnosed fibromyalgia of 4.3 per 1000 person-years, which, however, increased to 12 per 1000 person-years if a medical illness was present.

Key Points

- Patients with fibromyalgia suffer from a spectrum of associated symptoms that affect various body systems.
- Fibromyalgia affects 2–8% of the general population and is more common in women.
- Fibromyalgia can cause memory and concentration difficulties, also known as 'fibro-fog'.

References

1. Mayer EA, Bushnell MC. Functional pain syndromes. In: Mayer EA, Bushnell MC, Eds. *Functional pain syndromes: presentation and pathophysiology*, 1st ed. Seattle: International Association for the Study of Pain; 2009: pp. xv-xviii.

2. Clauw DJ. Fibromyalgia: a clinical review. *JAMA* 2014; 311(15): 1547-55.

3. Arthritis National Research Foundation. Fibromyalgia. Available from: https://curearthritis.org/fibromyalgia/?gclid=EAIaIQobChMI_tn9xOeA7gIVlu_tCh2QKgHVEAAYASAAEgI JSvD_BwE.

4.   Mandal A. Fibromyalgia epidemiology; 2019. Available from: https://www.news-medical.net/health/Fibromyalgia-Epidemiology.aspx.

5.   Walitt B, Nahin RL, Katz RS, *et al*. The prevalence and characteristics of fibromyalgia in the 2012 National Health Interview Survey. *PLoS ONE* 2015; 10(9): e0138024.

6.   Wolfe F. The epidemiology of fibromyalgia. *J Musculoskelet Pain* 1993; 1(3-4): 137-48.

7.   Creed F. A review of the incidence and risk factors for fibromyalgia and chronic widespread pain in population-based studies. *Pain* 2020; 161(6): 1169-76.

Chapter 3

Health economics and fibromyalgia

Introduction

Fibromyalgia imposes a huge economic burden in the context of both health and social care. Any medical illness involves direct costs (i.e. costs of investigation, treatment, care and rehabilitation of patients diagnosed with that particular illness), indirect costs (i.e. the value of economic losses in terms of work loss, lost productivity, disability and early mortality as a result of illness) and intangible costs (i.e. cost of pain and suffering due to illness) — see ▇ Figure 3.1 overleaf. In chronic conditions, it can be difficult to measure and estimate some of these costs. This chapter will discuss the health economic implications related to fibromyalgia.

Population statistics

It is estimated that 2–8% of the world's population are affected by fibromyalgia. While this may seem like a modest estimate, this equates to 200–400 million people worldwide who have the condition. One can thus appreciate the huge economic burden that fibromyalgia imposes on society.

According to the National Fibromyalgia Association, fibromyalgia costs the American economy between $12 and $14 billion annually, with a loss of overall productivity of 1–2%.

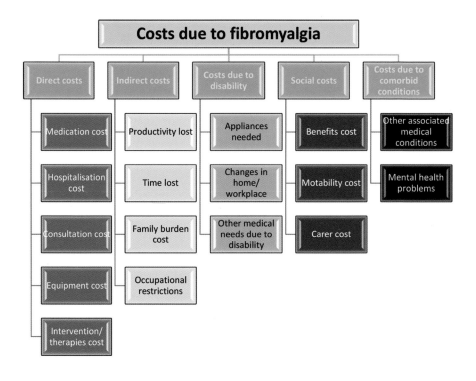

Figure 3.1. Costs related to fibromyalgia.

Further, the National Fibromyalgia & Chronic Pain Association in the United States reports that in 2012, more than 100 million Americans were affected by fibromyalgia, costing the national economy over $65 billion dollars.

Costs due to fibromyalgia

A survey in the USA of approximately 5000 patients with fibromyalgia found that the annual healthcare costs in this patient group (US$5945) was more than double the costs in the general population (US$2486). Using data from a US health insurance database covering 3 years, the authors found that the mean annual healthcare costs were three times higher among patients with fibromyalgia (US$9573), compared with non-fibromyalgia patients (US$3291), and median costs were five times higher. This study also found that the fibromyalgia group had a higher incidence of painful neuropathies, anxiety and depression, as well as higher use of analgesic pharmacotherapy, which could contribute to higher healthcare costs.

A Canadian study investigated a sample of 57 adults with fibromyalgia over 3 months and estimated an annual mean fibromyalgia-related cost of C$3804 per patient. The highest costs were incurred from purchase of medications, with an annual cost of C$1316, followed by costs of non-physician and physician consultations (C$516 and C$392 per year, respectively). Another Canadian study analysed data from a health insurance plan database of more than 16,000 patients with fibromyalgia, together with a control cohort of age- and gender-matched patients without fibromyalgia. This study found an annual cost of C$4065 for patients with fibromyalgia, compared with C$2766 for their non-fibromyalgia counterparts. Furthermore, results also showed the annual number of visits to physicians and physician's interventions was 25.1 for the fibromyalgia group and only 14.8 for the control group. A similar Canadian study using data from another health insurance plan database showed that mean annual healthcare costs associated with fibromyalgia were higher (a mean increase of C$493) than in the control group.

A Spanish study analysed medical records from a health provider database of more than 63,000 patients over 12 months. The authors found that costs in the fibromyalgia group were higher by €5010 than in the non-fibromyalgia group, after adjustment for other comorbidities. Annual drug expenditure per patient was also higher by €230 among patients with fibromyalgia patients, compared with control patients.

Other studies compared costs in fibromyalgia to costs related to other chronic rheumatological conditions. A Dutch study compared annual costs related to fibromyalgia to ankylosing spondylitis and found that average annual disease-related total societal costs per patient were €7813 for fibromyalgia, compared with €3205 for ankylosing spondylitis. This difference in costs could be explained by greater needs for formal and informal care, as well as for aids and adaptations, and by work days lost among patients with fibromyalgia. Well-being was lower in fibromyalgia (rating score 48) than in ankylosing spondylitis (rating score 67).

In summary, the costs and burden of fibromyalgia are clear, as demonstrated by the large number of international studies. It is evident that fibromyalgia is a condition that presents a huge socioeconomic challenge.

Indirect costs

Productivity costs among patients with fibromyalgia are related to time and productivity loss from paid and unpaid work due to pain caused by fibromyalgia, as well other illness-related factors.

A Canadian study showed that indirect costs could account for approximately 70% of the economic burden.

Costs due to disability

Evidence shows that the prevalence of disability among the working population with fibromyalgia is twice as high than disability due to other illnesses in the general working population. Costs are also high in those with fibromyalgia-associated disability.

Costs due to occupational restrictions

A Canadian study showed that in a sample of patients with fibromyalgia who had a paid job, an average of 5.6 days over a 3-month study period were lost due to pain. This is in contrast with an average of 25.1 days lost in household productivity over the same period among those with fibromyalgia who were unemployed due to pain related to their condition.

A work-related claims survey from the USA analysed approximately 5000 claims made by patients with fibromyalgia to calculate both direct and indirect costs associated with the condition. Results showed that for every US dollar spent on fibromyalgia-specific claims, employers spent approximately US$57–143 on additional direct and indirect costs.

A study from the United Kingdom was conducted over a decade ago on loss of work productivity among chronic fatigue patients who accessed specialist therapies alone, a group that constituted only a small proportion of the total population affected by fatigue. The study found a UK economy productivity loss of £75 million to £129 million, and these figures would certainly be higher if calculated in current times.

Out-of-pocket expenditure for patients

In 2012, the National Fibromyalgia Association carried out a survey among United States patients with fibromyalgia. The survey found that the average patient paid US$5310 annually for out-of-pocket treatment expenses. This included an annual average of US$1490 spent out-of-pocket on alternative modalities for pain management. Roughly equal amounts were also spent out-of-pocket on traditional and alternative care.

Relationship between disease severity and costs

Using the Fibromyalgia Impact Questionnaire (FIQ), a study showed that increased FIQ scores/disease severity correlated with higher annual costs (e.g. an increase in FIQ score from the sixth to seventh percentile resulted in an annual increase in costs of approximately US$865). Furthermore, the study showed that when the disease impact on the person was severe, even minimal increases in impact led to higher cost increments (compared with changes in the lower percentiles).

Furthermore, high pain scores were found to be associated with higher disease-related costs. Thus, a 1-point score increase on the Brief Pain Inventory resulted in an increase in annual costs of US$1453.

A Canadian study showed that comorbidity and disability among patients with fibromyalgia were significant contributors to direct costs in a multivariate analysis. The authors estimated that direct costs increased by approximately 20% with each additional comorbid condition.

Costs related to a concurrent diagnosis of fibromyalgia and depression

Both depression and fibromyalgia can be present concurrently, which imposes a significant economic burden. A study showed that mean costs were higher in patients diagnosed with both fibromyalgia and depression, compared with patients with either fibromyalgia or depression alone. Similarly, another study showed that total costs were significantly higher among patients with coexisting fibromyalgia and depression and/or anxiety, compared with those with fibromyalgia but without these symptoms.

Relationship between costs and early versus late treatment

A study from the USA looking at 33,470 newly diagnosed patients with fibromyalgia compared the costs among those who had early treatment versus those who had late treatment. Results showed total healthcare costs in the long term were significantly lower among those who received early treatment initiation, compared with late-treated patients (US$11,287 versus US$13,258, respectively, i.e. a 15% reduction). These findings strongly demonstrate significant cost savings associated with early treatment initiation.

A European study showed a reduction in costs following a diagnosis of fibromyalgia, compared with before a diagnosis of the condition is made. At 4 years after diagnosis, the costs reduced by £122.42 per year per patient, which was mainly as a result of a decrease in the use of investigations, followed by lower use of medications. This retrospective study included patients with a recorded diagnosis of fibromyalgia from 1998 and analysed data up to 10 years before and up to 4 years after the index date. It is assumed that the cost savings would be significantly improved in current times.

Fibromyalgia is not only a medical disease, but also a significant socioeconomic burden. Policymakers, politicians, healthcare managers and clinical professionals should work together with patients suffering from fibromyalgia to look at streamlining pathways for better management of this condition, with the overall aim of saving taxpayers' money and easing patient suffering.

Key Points

- Evidence from international studies shows that fibromyalgia is a significant economic burden.
- Indirect costs are likely to account for the majority of the costs but are more difficult to quantify accurately.
- Comorbid conditions and depression significantly increase fibromyalgia-related costs.
- Early diagnosis of fibromyalgia contributes to significant cost savings, mainly due to reduced use of investigations and medications.

References

1. National Fibromyalgia Association. Fibromyalgia: the economic burden. Available from: https://www.fmaware.org/fibromyalgia-the-economic-burden/.

2. Collin SM, Crawley E, May MT, et al. The impact of CFS/ME on employment and productivity in the UK: a cross-sectional study based on the CFS/ME national outcomes database. BMC Health Serv Res 2011; 11: 217.

3. Fibromyalgia news today; 2015. Study assesses economic burden of fibromyalgia in the US. Available from: https://fibromyalgianewstoday.com/2015/06/04/study-assesses-economic-burden-fibromyalgia-us/.

4. Berger A, Dukes E, Martin S, et al. Characteristics and healthcare costs of patients with fibromyalgia syndrome. Int J Clin Pract 2007; 61(9): 1498-508.

5. Lachaine J, Beauchemin C, Landry PA. Clinical and economic characteristics of patients with fibromyalgia syndrome. Clin J Pain 2010; 26(4): 284-90.

6.   White KP, Speechley M, Harth M, Ostbye T. The London Fibromyalgia Epidemiology Study: direct health care costs of fibromyalgia syndrome in London, Canada. *J Rheumatol* 1999; 26(4): 885-9.

7.   Penrod JR, Bernatsky S, Adam V, *et al.* Health services costs and their determinants in women with fibromyalgia. *J Rheumatol* 2004; 31(7): 1391-8.

8.   Robinson RL, Birnbaum HG, Morley MA, *et al.* Economic cost and epidemiological characteristics of patients with fibromyalgia claims. *J Rheumatol* 2003; 30(6): 1318-25.

9.   Robinson RL, Birnbaum HG, Morley MA, *et al.* Depression and fibromyalgia: treatment and cost when diagnosed separately or concurrently. *J Rheumatol* 2004; 31(8): 1621-9.

10.   Lacasse A, Bourgault P, Choinière M. Fibromyalgia-related costs and loss of productivity: a substantial social burden. *BMC Musculoskelet Disord* 2016; 17: 168.

11.   Sicras-Mainar A, Rejas J, Navarro R, *et al.* Treating patients with fibromyalgia in primary care settings under routine medical practice: a claim database cost and burden of illness study. *Arthritis Res Ther* 2009; 11(2): R54.

12.   Boonen A, van den Heuvel R, van Tubergen A, *et al.* Large differences in cost of illness and wellbeing between patients with fibromyalgia, chronic low back pain, or ankylosing spondylitis. *Ann Rheum Dis* 2005; 64(3): 396-402.

13.   Frech F, Qian C, Gore M, *et al.* Cost implications of early treatment initiation among patients with newly diagnosed fibromyalgia. *Am J Pharm Benefits* 2017; 9: 200-7.

14.   Wolfe F, Aarflot T, Bruusgaard D, *et al.* Fibromyalgia and disability: report on the Moss International Working Group on medico-legal aspects of chronic widespread musculoskeletal pain complaints and fibromyalgia. *Scand J Rheumatol* 1995; 24(2): 112-8.

15.   Annemans L, Wessely S, Spaepen E, *et al.* Health economic consequences related to the diagnosis of fibromyalgia syndrome. *Arthritis Rheum* 2008; 58(3): 895-902.

Chapter 4

Prognosis of fibromyalgia

Introduction

Approximately 2% of the general population have fibromyalgia, while the condition affects up to 20% of rheumatology patients. It can be difficult to distinguish between fibromyalgia and other functional pain syndromes. Treatments for fibromyalgia have limited efficacy and the overall prognosis is considered poor.

Prognosis

Numerous studies have clearly demonstrated that fibromyalgia is not an organ-threatening disease and is not associated with increased overall mortality.

Fibromyalgia is a chronic condition. However, once its diagnosis is confirmed, overall well-being and pain scores tend to improve, as shown in many epidemiological studies.

Long-term follow-up studies from the USA have suggested that patients with fibromyalgia have an average of ten outpatient visits every year and one hospitalisation every 3 years.

There is a risk of relapse and flare-up in the disease course and, therefore, patients with fibromyalgia should be educated on maintaining a healthy lifestyle and the need to keep active, as well as on coping and pacing strategies. Symptoms can be significantly improved if ongoing stressors are relieved and pain management is adequate.

Fibromyalgia is associated with an increased risk of disability. However, many experts prefer to refrain from labelling patients with fibromyalgia as being disabled, as this can frequently result in worsening of symptoms and hamper their recovery pathway.

Outcomes

A six-centre longitudinal study from the USA investigated the functional outcomes of fibromyalgia in patients seen in rheumatology centres over 7 years. Results showed that functional disability worsened slightly over time, with pain, fatigue, sleep disturbance, anxiety and depression remaining unchanged, whereas health satisfaction improved slightly. The authors concluded that values at the first assessment are predictive of final values. This study highlights poor outcomes in established fibromyalgia and the need for treatments to be tailored to individual patients.

Different studies have described outcomes in patients with fibromyalgia ranging from poor to moderate. A German study showed that a multimodal therapeutic approach should be tailored to individual patients and even then, in many cases, the prognosis is only moderately successful.

A Swiss prospective 6-year follow-up study of a cohort of patients with fibromyalgia showed that symptoms persisted over the study period. However, these patients were able to cope with their symptoms and their quality of life improved over this time.

Diagnosis of fibromyalgia: to have or not to have

The question of whether having a diagnosis of fibromyalgia is beneficial or not remains a subject of constant debate. A systematic review of studies conducted in different countries found no evidence that having a fibromyalgia diagnosis would contribute to a poor prognosis. Of note, there is moderate-to-good quality evidence showing that a diagnosis of fibromyalgia can reduce the use of healthcare resources by patients suffering from the condition.

Effects of fibromyalgia treatment

A 2013 study from Indianapolis showed that patients with fibromyalgia who received treatment over 12 months showed modest improvements in four health outcomes and patient satisfaction, despite high use of resources and medications. Other outcome measures included visits to outpatient care, missed days of work and days of care by unpaid caregivers.

Pain scores and outcomes

A longitudinal study of patients with fibromyalgia in the USA reported improved function and sleep over a 2-year follow-up. Patients who achieved ≥2-point improvement in pain scores experienced greater improvement in these two outcome measures.

Outcomes in specialised clinics

A French systematic review showed poor overall outcomes in patients with fibromyalgia. Of note, outcomes outside specialised clinics might be better, as these clinics manage patients with significant abnormal illness behaviours.

Outcomes in the community

An Australian study reported that fibromyalgia managed in the community carried a better prognosis. The study showed 24.2% of patients with fibromyalgia went into remission over a 2-year follow-up period. Regular physical exercise, rather than pharmacotherapy, correlated with improved outcomes. These results indicate that simple interventions may be associated with better outcomes in a significant number of patients with fibromyalgia who are managed in the community.

Key Points

- Fibromyalgia is a long-term disease, with symptoms that can be well controlled.
- Having an early diagnosis of fibromyalgia can help in reducing use of healthcare resources.
- Fibromyalgia does not contribute to an increased risk of mortality or organ damage.

References

1. Driver CB. Fibromyalgia; 2020. Available from: https://www.medicinenet.com/fibromyalgia_facts/article.htm.

2. Boomershine CS. What is the prognosis of fibromyalgia?; 2020. Available from: https://www.medscape.com/answers/329838-18848/what-is-the-prognosis-of-fibromyalgia.

3. Wolfe F, Anderson J, Harkness D, *et al.* Health status and disease severity in fibromyalgia. Results of a six-center longitudinal study. *Arthritis Rheum* 1997; 40(9): 1571-9.

4. Schwarz VM, Kapfhammer HP. The fibromyalgia syndrome. *MMW Fortschr Med* 2004; 146(29-30): 34-7.

5. Baumgartner E, Finckh A, Cedraschi C, Vischer TL. A six year prospective study of a cohort of patients with fibromyalgia. *Ann Rheum Dis* 2002; 61(7): 644-5.

6. Schaefer CP, Adams EH, Udall M, *et al.* Fibromyalgia outcomes over time: results from a prospective observational study in the United States. *Open Rheumatol J* 2016; 10: 109-21.

7. Robinson RL, Kroenke K, Williams DA, *et al.* Longitudinal observation of treatment patterns and outcomes for patients with fibromyalgia: 12-month findings from the reflections study. *Pain Med* 2013; 14(9): 1400-15.

8. Cathébras P, Lauwers A, Rousset H. [Fibromyalgia. A critical review]. *Ann Med Interne (Paris)* 1998; 149(7): 406-14.

9. Granges G, Zilko P, Littlejohn GO. Fibromyalgia syndrome: assessment of the severity of the condition 2 years after diagnosis. *J Rheumatol* 1994; 21(3): 523-9.

Section 2

Causes of fibromyalgia

Fibromyalgia

Chapter 5

Aetiopathogenesis of fibromyalgia

Introduction

The exact cause of fibromyalgia still remains unclear. Various theories have been proposed, which will be discussed in Chapters 6–10. Whether fibromyalgia should be considered as primarily a muscular, neurogenic, endocrine or psychiatric disorder has been the subject of intense debate over the years, whereas various theories involving other body systems in the pathophysiology of fibromyalgia have also been suggested.

Primary or secondary disease

In many patients, fibromyalgia can occur without a primary cause. Patients can be diagnosed with fibromyalgia secondary to other diseases, including rheumatological, neurological or psychiatric disorders, infection and diabetes — see █ Figure 5.1 overleaf.

Aetiopathogenesis

Is fibromyalgia caused by a muscle disorder — the 'muscle theory'?

Given that muscle pain and fatigue are the main symptoms of fibromyalgia, localised muscle pathology was previously considered by

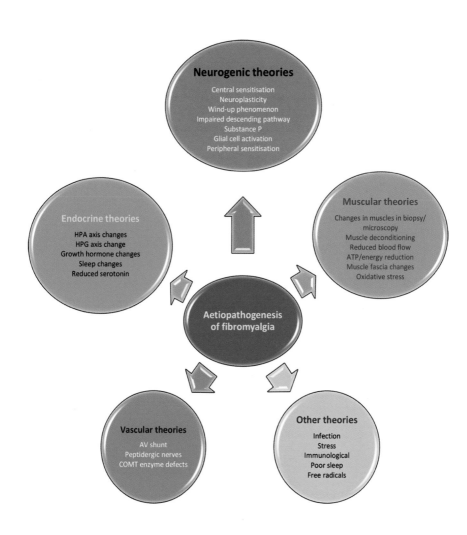

Figure 5.1. Aetiopathogenesis of fibromyalgia. ATP = adenosine triphosphate; COMT = catechol-O-methyltransferase; HPA = hypothalamic-pituitary-adrenal; HPG = hypothalamic-pituitary-gonadal.

scientists as the aetiological factor. However, given the evidence of central sensitisation that occurs in fibromyalgia, it is now clear that the aetiology of this condition is more complex than can be explained by only one causative factor (see Chapters 6-10).

Is fibromyalgia caused by a neurogenic disorder — the 'neurogenic theory'?

Changes in neurotransmitter levels in the brain, spinal cord and nerves, modulating the pain pathway, have been proposed as an aetiological factor in fibromyalgia. Sensitisation of the nervous system can occur both centrally and peripherally in fibromyalgia. Persistent peripheral pain stimulation can result in central sensitisation and chronicity of this painful condition. This will be discussed in detail in Chapter 6.

Is fibromyalgia caused by an endocrine disorder — the 'endocrine theory'?

Hormonal changes can play a role in the pathophysiology of fibromyalgia. In particular, changes to the hypothalamic-pituitary-adrenal (HPA) axis, as well as changes in growth hormone levels, have been reported in many studies. This will be discussed in detail in Chapter 8.

Is fibromyalgia caused by a vascular disorder — the 'vascular theory'?

Scientists have proposed that innervation of arteriole-venule shunts could explain the chronicity of fibromyalgia. Global serotonin dysregulation has also been suggested as a vascular factor underlying the aetiopathogenesis of fibromyalgia. This will be discussed in detail in Chapter 9.

Other possible aetiological factors

- Genetic factors: inherited from parents.
- Environmental factors: triggered by physically or emotionally stressful events or trauma.
- Infections predisposing to the condition.
- Immunological factors.

- Nutritional factors.
- Psychosocial factors.
- Disordered sleep.

These will be discussed in detail in Chapter 10.

Multisymptom disorder based on stress system dysregulation

A simplistic approach to understanding the aetiology of fibromyalgia is to consider it as a condition of excessive stress following a prolonged period of physical and/or emotional stress. This could easily explain the symptoms affecting multiple body systems such as sensory pain problems, physical problems, fatigue, emotional problems and neurocognitive deficits, including 'brain fog'.

It is easier to consider fibromyalgia as a condition caused by an interplay of neural, neurohormonal and immunological causative mechanisms. A prolonged history of psychosocial stress (including abuse or trauma) and specific personality traits, such as maladaptive behaviours, are seen as predisposing factors.

Multiple factors

This book contains six chapters focused on the aetiopathogenesis of fibromyalgia syndrome. It is clear that the aetiology of fibromyalgia cannot be explained by one single causative factor. It is in the author's opinion that chronicity of fibromyalgia is the result of a combination of neurological, muscular and endocrine pathologies, against a background of triggering factors, including trauma or a psychological event, especially in genetically predisposed individuals with poor coping abilities.

Key Points

- No single causative factor can solely explain the aetiopathogenesis of fibromyalgia.
- Central and peripheral sensitisation occurs in fibromyalgia patients.
- A combination of various factors, together with poor coping abilities, will result in chronicity of fibromyalgia.

References

1. Bellato E, Marini E, Castoldi F, *et al*. Fibromyalgia syndrome: etiology, pathogenesis, diagnosis, and treatment. *Pain Res Treat* 2012; 2012: 426130.

2. Ablin JN, Buskila D, Van Houdenhove B, *et al*. Is fibromyalgia a discrete entity? *Autoimmun Rev* 2012; 11(8): 585-8.

3. Albrecht PJ, Hou Q, Argoff CE, *et al*. Excessive peptidergic sensory innervation of cutaneous arteriole-venule shunts (AVS) in the palmar glabrous skin of fibromyalgia patients: implications of widespread deep tissue pain and fatigue. *Pain Med* 2013; 14(6): 895-915.

4. Amin OA, Abouzeid SM, Ali SA, *et al*. Clinical association of vitamin D and serotonin levels among patients with fibromyalgia syndrome. *Neuropsychiatr Dis Treat* 2019; 15: 1421-6.

Chapter 6

Neurogenic theories

Introduction

Although various aetiological mechanisms have been suggested, many groups have proposed a neurogenic aetiopathogenic mechanism underlying fibromyalgia. Support for a neurogenic mechanism comes from clinical practice in which improved outcomes are observed in patients with fibromyalgia treated with neuropathic medications and other interventions.

Central sensitisation

Repeated stimulation of the central nervous system causes an increased response to this stimulation in some patients — a phenomenon termed central sensitisation. Central sensitisation can be due to various reasons, including, but not limited to, the following:

- Repeated stimulation causing spontaneous ectopic neuronal activity.
- Enlarged receptive fields on stimulation.
- Augmented responses in primary afferent fibres.
- 'Wind-up' phenomenon: increased excitability of spinal cord neurons with temporal summation of pain, whereby following a painful stimulus, subsequent stimuli produce a higher response, with C-fibres and N-methyl-D-aspartate (NMDA) receptors in the post-synaptic membrane in the spinal dorsal horn suggested as potentiators of 'wind-up'.

- Neuroplasticity: changes in nerve conduction and modulation causing more intense signals.
- Inflammatory changes causing excitation of dorsal horn neurons.
- Abnormal temporal summation of pain.
- Abnormal activation of pain-related brain areas.

Nociceptive stimuli release a variety of chemical neurotransmitters, including serotonin, prostaglandins, leukotrienes, substance P and calcitonin gene-related peptide (CGRP). These neurochemicals sensitise peripheral C-fibres (causing peripheral sensitisation) and spinal cord neurons (causing central sensitisation). Both peripheral and central sensitisation lead to amplified nociceptive input, which, in turn, results in enlarged peripheral receptive fields with increased dorsal horn excitability.

Spinal cord and brain plasticity

Injury to peripheral tissue or nerves causes hyperalgesia or allodynia, which is the perception of pain to stimuli such as light touch. When this results in hyperexcitability in the central nervous system, it is referred to as plasticity. The production of axonal sprouts that are sensitive to light touch/painful stimuli has been proposed as a mechanism underlying plasticity. Spontaneous discharges from these axonal sprouts and dorsal root ganglia increase neuronal barrage into the central nervous system, causing increased pain.

Descending pain pathways

Various theories have proposed that impairment in the descending inhibitory pain pathways causes increased central sensitisation.

Substance P

Substance P is a nociceptive neurotransmitter present in the dorsal horn. High concentrations of both substance P and nerve growth factor (NGF) have been found in the cerebrospinal fluid (CSF) in patients with fibromyalgia. The concentration of N-terminal peptide of substance P has been found to be twice higher in patients with fibromyalgia, compared with the general population.

There is also evidence of low concentrations of Met-enkephalin-Arg-Phe in fibromyalgia. Further research is needed in this area.

Regional cerebral blood flow variations

In patients with fibromyalgia, regional cerebral blood flow (rCBF) is significantly lower in the caudate nucleus and thalamus, both of which are involved in signalling the presence of noxious events. It has been proposed that low rCBF could be the cause of abnormal pain perception. Low rCBF could be considered a marker of impaired inhibition of nociceptive transmission at the caudate and thalamic level in the pain neuromatrix.

Chemical imbalances in the brain

Serotonin, noradrenaline and dopamine are hormones known to play important roles in regulating mood, sleep, appetite, behaviour and response to stressful situations. Research has shown low levels of these hormones in the brain of patients with fibromyalgia, suggesting a causal link to the condition.

Dysfunction in the monoaminergic system in neurons has been suggested to be the main pathological mechanism in fibromyalgia. Studies have shown elevated levels of neurotransmitters, including glutamate and substance P, in fibromyalgia, whereas decreased levels of serotonin and noradrenaline in the spinal cord in descending anti-nociceptive pathways have been observed. Other chemical changes in the central nervous system include dopamine dysregulation and altered activity of endogenous opioids in the brain.

Glial cell activation

Activated glial cells have been found to maintain exaggerated pain states, suggesting that glial cell activation could underlie fibromyalgia.

Immunohistochemical studies have indicated that spinal cord microglia and astrocytes could play a role in causing painful conditions.

Glial cell activation caused by painful stimuli can release proinflammatory cytokines, prostaglandins, nitric oxide and reactive oxygen species. These, in turn, can stimulate and prolong spinal cord hyperexcitability.

Peripheral pathways

Changes in receptors in the nociceptor system in skin and muscles have been suggested to be responsible for causing abnormal pain sensations in fibromyalgia.

Various receptor changes have been proposed, including:

● Sensitisation of vanilloid receptors.
● Changes in acid-sensing ion channel receptors.
● Changes in purino-receptors.

Tissue mediators of inflammation and NGF could contribute to these receptor changes, thus stimulating the pain pathway.

Abnormalities in the peripheral nervous system could also contribute to increased nociceptive tonic stimulation in the spinal cord, which could lead to central sensitisation.

Peripheral nociceptive dysregulation

Skin biopsies in patients with fibromyalgia have shown reduced numbers of epidermal nerve fibres, whereas microneurography studies have demonstrated increased peripheral sensitisation.

Neuroimaging in elucidating the aetiopathogenesis of fibromyalgia

Functional neuroimaging has enabled researchers to have a better understanding of the causation of fibromyalgia, as shown below:

- Single-photon emission computed tomography (SPECT): infusion of a radioactive tracer showed reduced rCBF in the thalamus and caudate nucleus.
- Positron emission tomography (PET): has higher temporal and spatial resolution, compared with SPECT. Changes in blood flow relates to increased processing of subnoxious somatosensory signals and impaired cognitive processing in fibromyalgia.
- Functional magnetic resonance imaging (fMRI): has higher temporal and spatial resolution, compared with PET or SPECT. Studies using fMRI showed augmented central pain processing and changes in the descending inhibitory pain system, which explains the increased response to painful stimuli in patients with fibromyalgia.

fMRI studies in fibromyalgia

fMRI studies have provided evidence of central neuronal alteration in nociceptive and nociplastic processes in fibromyalgia. Identical stimuli produced greater neuronal activation in pain processing areas in patients with fibromyalgia, compared with the control group. Furthermore, greater neuronal activity has been observed in wider areas, including the posterior insula and the secondary somatosensory cortex.

fMRI enables determination of connectivity between various areas of the brain in both resting and active periods. There is greater connectivity between a network called the 'default mode network' (that is, active when the brain is at rest) and the insula (nociceptive area) in patients with fibromyalgia. By contrast, hypoconnectivity has been shown in anti-nociceptive areas of the brain in patients with fibromyalgia.

The neuromatrix theory

The neuromatrix theory was elaborated in detail by V. S. Ramachandran in the setting of phantom limbs. The theory has many applicable concepts that could help in understanding chronic pain conditions such as fibromyalgia. Systematic psychosocial testing and functional imaging have shown neural plasticity in the adult human brain. By tracking these perceptual changes (referred sensations) and changes in the cortical topography, scientists explored how the activity of sensory maps gives rise to conscious experience. This allows study of the intersensory effects and the manner in which the brain constructs and updates a 'body image' throughout life.

The same principles could be applied to patients with fibromyalgia. In fibromyalgia, it is possible that a simple trauma or injury could result in changes in the neuromatrix output in a systemic manner, rather than in a localised pattern. This could explain the widespread dysaesthesia in patients with fibromyalgia that could not be otherwise explained simply by one peripheral or central pain theory as causation of the condition.

In the above-mentioned review, the neuromatrix theory is proposed as the most plausible explanation for fibromyalgia, which can be applied practically, with successful outcomes, in the rehabilitation of patients with fibromyalgia. In another subsequent review by Moseley, two fundamental principles were suggested to explain this approach based on the neuromatrix theory:

- Pain is the brain output when the brain concludes that the body tissue is in danger and action is needed.
- Pain is a multisystem output produced when an individual-specific cortical pain neuromatrix is activated.

While the first principle can be easily applied to acute pain scenarios, the second principle provides a valid scientific basis to explain chronic pain conditions such as fibromyalgia.

Chronicity in the neuromatrix theory

The neuromatrix theory proposes that enhanced sensitivity of the pain neuromatrix (due to increased synaptic efficacy) means that less input is required for activation of the neuromatrix. Smaller and less relevant inputs are sufficient to activate the neuromatrix and cause pain. Even simple movements that are not supposed to be painful or just seeing another person perform painful movements can cause pain. This explains the difficulty faced by patients with fibromyalgia with justifying or proving their pain to other people, including their family or healthcare professionals.

Neurosignature

The neuromatrix is created by a multidimensional experience produced by characteristic 'neurosignature' patterns that are determined by various factors, including, but not limited to: presenting trauma, persisting inflammation, genetic predisposition, memory or previous experiences, environmental influences, stress and psychological contributors and behavioural patterns including catastrophisation. These are modified by sensory experience, as well as by a widely distributed neural network termed the 'body-self neuromatrix'. These neurosignatures change continuously with bombarding inputs from the various factors mentioned above, resulting in a continuously evolving neuromatrix throughout the fibromyalgia patient's life.

Key Points

- Central sensitisation occurs in fibromyalgia due to various changes in the pain pathway.
- Hyperexcitability of the central nervous system due to plasticity causes allodynia and dysaesthesia.
- Chemical imbalances in the brain and glial cell activation have been found to occur in fibromyalgia.
- Supporting evidence for the neurogenic theory involving pain pathways to explain the aetiopathogenesis of fibromyalgia have come from fMRI studies.
- The neuromatrix theory is easily applicable clinically to explain fibromyalgia and engage patients in their recovery pathway.

References

1. Bellato E, Marini E, Castoldi F, *et al.* Fibromyalgia syndrome: etiology, pathogenesis, diagnosis, and treatment. *Pain Res Treat* 2012; 2012: 426130.
2. Staud R, Smitherman ML. Peripheral and central sensitization in fibromyalgia: pathogenetic role. *Curr Pain Headache Rep* 2002; 6(4): 259-66.
3. Pillemer SR, Bradley LA, Crofford LJ, *et al.* The neuroscience and endocrinology of fibromyalgia. *Arthritis Rheum* 1997; 40(11): 1928-39.
4. Siracusa R, Di Paola RD, Cuzzocrea S, Impellizzeri D. Fibromyalgia: pathogenesis, mechanisms, diagnosis and treatment options update. *Int J Mol Sci* 2021; 22(8): 3891.
5. Doppler K, Rittner HL, Deckart M, Sommer C. Reduced dermal nerve fiber diameter in skin biopsies of patients with fibromyalgia. *Pain* 2015; 156(11): 2319-25.
6. NHS. Causes: fibromyalgia; 2019. Available from: https://www.nhs.uk/conditions/fibromyalgia/causes/.
7. Watkins LR, Milligan ED, Maier SF. Spinal cord glia: new players in pain. *Pain* 2001; 93(3): 201-5.
8. Napadow V, Kim J, Clauw DJ, Harris RE. Decreased intrinsic brain connectivity is associated with reduced clinical pain in fibromyalgia. *Arthritis Rheum* 2012; 64(7): 2398-403.
9. Ramachandran VS, Rogers-Ramachandran D. Phantom limbs and neural plasticity. *Arch Neurol* 2000; 57(3): 317-20.
10. Moseley GL. A pain neuromatrix approach to patients with chronic pain. *Man Ther* 2003; 8(3): 130-40.
11. Melzack R. Evolution of the neuromatrix theory of pain. The Prithvi Raj Lecture: presented at the third World Congress of World Institute of Pain, Barcelona 2004. *Pain Pract* 2005; 5(2): 85-94.

Chapter 7

Myogenic theories

Introduction

As muscle pain and fatigue are the main symptoms in patients with fibromyalgia, all initial research studies only focused on muscle problems as the aetiology of the disease. However, chronic pain conditions such as fibromyalgia are too complex to be explained by a simple aetiopathological theory. Focusing on a biopsychosocial model will help in patient recovery from fibromyalgia, although appropriate metaphors can be used to help explain the need to maintain muscle tonicity and adopt pacing strategies (these are discussed in Chapter 24).

Pathological muscle abnormalities

Various pathological muscle abnormalities have been documented in patients with fibromyalgia, including ragged red fibres, rubber band-like morphology, decreased capillary bed in muscles, thickened endothelium and sarcolemmal membrane damage. However, none of these can be consistently detected or linked to the clinical symptoms in all patients with fibromyalgia.

Histochemical and light and electron microscopy investigations carried out in muscle biopsy samples of patients with fibromyalgia found type II fibre atrophy, a moth-eaten appearance in type I fibres, segmental muscle fibre necrosis, lipid and glycogen deposition and subsarcolemmal mitochondrial accumulation in a majority of these patients. In summary, there are definite, although non-specific, histological changes in muscles, which are suspected to be due to chronic muscle spasm or ischaemia of unknown aetiology.

Another study showed abnormal rubber band-like structures and interconnecting networks of reticular or elastic fibres in muscle biopsy samples taken from patients with fibromyalgia. This study also found reduced phosphate levels in muscle cells. However, these findings are not specific to, and not diagnostic of, fibromyalgia.

Muscle fatigue and hyperalgesia

Animal models of non-inflammatory pain, in which acidic saline is repeatedly injected into the gastrocnemius muscle, have been shown to reproduce clinical signs and symptoms of fibromyalgia. Studies using these animal models found that fatigue can increase the risk of developing hyperalgesia to even mild insult. These findings can help to clarify the association between fatigue and chronic pain.

Muscle deconditioning

Muscle deconditioning was proposed in the 1990s as the cause of fibromyalgia. However, it has since become clear that muscle deconditioning occurs in a variety of chronic pain conditions that cannot be explained by muscle-related causes alone. It is a 'chicken and egg' debate, as muscle deconditioning and wasting can equally develop as a sequela of chronic pain itself.

Reduced muscle blood flow

One study estimated aerobic fitness in patients with fibromyalgia, compared with controls, by determining exercising blood flow with the use of xenon-133 clearance measurements. The authors found reduced xenon-133 clearance in patients with fibromyalgia, and proposed a 'detraining phenomenon' in muscles as the cause of fibromyalgia. However, subsequent studies have not reproduced these results.

ATP reserves in muscles

Adenosine triphosphate (ATP) levels indicate the energy reserve in a cell. Histochemical studies of muscle biopsies taken from patients with fibromyalgia using the muscle enzyme ATPase have shown low ATP levels, indicating low energy reserve.

Some scientists have proposed that fibromyalgia could be caused by an 'energy crisis' at the cellular level in muscles. However, research studies have not been consistent in showing localised defects in muscle metabolism. Studies using maximum rate of oxygen uptake (VO_2max) in muscles and phosphorus (^{31}P) magnetic resonance spectroscopy have concluded that energy crisis or depletion is not specific to fibromyalgia, as it has also been seen in sedentary individuals.

Pathology in muscle fascia

Some authors have proposed that a dysfunction of intramuscular connective tissue, or fascia, could explain the development of fibromyalgia. Immunohistochemical staining showed increased levels of collagen and inflammatory mediators in the connective tissue surrounding muscle cells in fibromyalgia. Anatomically, the fascia is richly innervated, and fibroblasts in the fascia are known to secrete proinflammatory cytokines, including interleukin-6, in response to stress. It is hypothesised that these inflammatory changes could lead to central sensitisation in fibromyalgia.

Low intramuscular collagen content

A study measuring collagen concentration in muscle biopsies from patients with fibromyalgia found that the fibromyalgia group had lower concentrations of hydroxyproline and major amino acids of collagen, compared with the control group. There was no change in concentration of the major amino acids of myosin or of total protein. The study concluded that patients with fibromyalgia had significantly lower amounts of intramuscular collagen.

Reduced micro-circulation in the muscles

Studies using light microscopy of muscle biopsies from patients with fibromyalgia showed a reduced number of capillaries per square millimetre.

Scientists have proposed that pain in fibromyalgia could be due to low-level ischaemia and its metabolic sequelae induced by vasomotor dysregulation. Vasodilatory factors, including exercise, can relieve pain in fibromyalgia by increasing muscle perfusion.

Ischaemic change in muscle can produce an inflammatory systemic response whereby interleukin-1 beta (IL-1β) activates its receptor, increasing the expression of acid-sensing ion channel 3 (ASIC3). This, in turn, induces the c-Jun N-terminal kinase (JNK) signalling pathway and modulates afferent impulses, thereby reducing the pain threshold.

Intramuscular adiposity in fibromyalgia

Increased intramuscular adiposity, along with reduced mitochondrial density and function, has been observed in fibromyalgia. Animal studies have shown that adipose tissue secretes proinflammatory cytokines that contribute to perpetuating pain. Further research in human trials are awaited to ascertain the role of adipose tissue in fibromyalgia.

Oxidative stress and free radicals in muscles

Vascular hypoperfusion in muscles stimulates production of inducible nitric oxide synthase (iNOS), an enzyme involved in nitric oxide synthesis. High levels of nitric oxide can lead to cellular oxidative stress, which has been shown to contribute to exertional fatigue in fibromyalgia. Furthermore, stimulation of nitric oxide leads to increased micro-dialysate lactate in fibromyalgia, with more suppressive effects of nitric oxide on oxidative phosphorylation found in patients with fibromyalgia.

Mitochondrial dysfunction

Studies have shown the role of mitochondria in oxidative stress causing fibromyalgia. Deficiency in the antioxidant coenzyme Q10 alters mitochondrial function, resulting in increased generation of reactive oxygen species in fibromyalgia.

Reduced enzymes in muscles

Reduced muscle levels of the oxidative enzymes 3-hydroxyacyl-CoA dehydrogenase and citrate synthase were demonstrated in patients with fibromyalgia. These reduced enzyme levels could indicate reduced physical activity, rather than be a cause per se of fibromyalgia.

Motor control failure: central or peripheral?

Surface electromyography was used to study muscle fatigue that was evoked by voluntary and involuntary (electrically caused) contractions in patients with fibromyalgia. It was found that the motor recruitment pattern during voluntary contractions was altered, with fewer myoelectrical manifestations of fatigue, in the fibromyalgia group. The authors concluded that fibromyalgia is probably more related to central motor control failure than to peripheral muscle membrane alterations.

Limitations of the muscle pathology model

Muscle abnormalities observed in microscopy studies are not consistently detected, and the results are not reproducible across all studies of patients with fibromyalgia. Furthermore, these abnormalities do not always correlate with symptoms and clinical presentations of fibromyalgia, thus suggesting a multimodal pathogenesis that leads to central sensitisation in the disease. However, knowledge of the aetiopathogenesis underlying the 'muscle theory' will help inform mechanism-based treatments in fibromyalgia in a more effective manner.

Key Points

- Microscopic changes in muscle fibres have been extensively documented in patients with fibromyalgia, although these are neither consistent nor reproducible; these changes do not correlate directly with the clinical presentation of fibromyalgia.
- Reduced muscle blood flow, reduced ATP, mitochondrial dysfunction and oxidative stress are a few of the underlying mechanisms proposed in the aetiology of fibromyalgia.
- Recent research has focused on muscle fascia and adipose tissue as possible causes of pain in fibromyalgia.
- Many scientists have put forward theories of microscopic muscle changes, while suggesting that these abnormalities lead to central sensitisation via different pathways in fibromyalgia.

References

1. Staud R, Domingo MA. Evidence for abnormal pain processing in fibromyalgia syndrome. *Pain Med* 2001; 2(3): 208-15.

2. Kalyan-Raman UP, Kalyan-Raman K, Yunus MB, Masi AT. Muscle pathology in primary fibromyalgia syndrome: a light microscopic, histochemical and ultrastructural study. *J Rheumatol* 1984; 11(6): 808-13.

3. Yunus MB, Kalyan-Raman UP. Muscle biopsy findings in primary fibromyalgia and other forms of nonarticular rheumatism. *Rheum Dis Clin North Am* 1989; 15(1): 115-34.

4.   Yokoyama T, Lisi TL, Moore SA, Sluka KA. Muscle fatigue increases the probability of developing hyperalgesia in mice. *J Pain* 2007; 8(9): 692-9.

5.   Lindman R, Eriksson A, Thornell LE. Fiber type composition of the human female trapezius muscle: enzyme-histochemical characteristics. *Am J Anat* 1991; 190(4): 385-92.

6.   Simms RW, Roy SH, Hrovat M, *et al.* Lack of association between fibromyalgia syndrome and abnormalities in muscle energy metabolism. *Arthritis Rheum* 1994; 37(6): 794-800.

7.   Klemp P, Nielsen HV, Korsgård J, Crone P. Blood flow in fibromyotic muscles. *Scand J Rehabil Med* 1982; 14(2): 81-2.

8.   Bennett RM, Clark SR, Goldberg L, *et al.* Aerobic fitness in patients with fibrositis. A controlled study of respiratory gas exchange and 133xenon clearance from exercising muscle. *Arthritis Rheum* 1989; 32(4): 454-60.

9.   Liptan GL. Fascia: a missing link in our understanding of the pathology of fibromyalgia. *J Bodyw Mov Ther* 2010; 14(1): 3-12.

10.   Gronemann ST, Ribel-Madsen S, Bartels EM, *et al.* Collagen and muscle pathology in fibromyalgia patients. *Rheumatology (Oxford)* 2004; 43(1): 27-31.

11.   Lindh M, Johansson G, Hedberg M, *et al.* Muscle fiber characteristics, capillaries and enzymes in patients with fibromyalgia and controls. *Scand J Rheumatol* 1995; 24(1): 34-7.

12.   Katz DL, Greene L, Ali A, Faridi Z. The pain of fibromyalgia syndrome is due to muscle hypoperfusion induced by regional vasomotor dysregulation. *Med Hypo* 2007; 69(3): 517-25.

13.   Ross JL, Queme LF, Cohen ER, *et al.* Muscle IL 1 drives ischaemic myalgia via ASIC3-mediated sensory neuron sensitization. *J Neurosci* 2016; 36(26): 6857-71.

14.   Bordoni B, Marelli F, Morabito B, *et al.* Fascial preadipocytes: another missing pieces of the puzzle to understand fibromyalgia? *Open Access Rheumatol* 2018; 10: 27-32.

15.   McIver KL, Evans C, Kraus RM, *et al.* NO-mediated alterations in skeletal muscle nutritive blood flow and lactate metabolism in fibromyalgia. *Pain* 2006; 120(1-2): 161-9.

16.   Cordero MD, de Miguel M, Carmona-López I, *et al.* Oxidative stress and mitochondrial dysfunction in fibromyalgia. *Neuro Endocrinol Lett* 2010; 31(2): 169-73.

17.   Casale R, Sarzi-Puttini P, Atzeni F, *et al.* Central motor control failure in fibromyalgia: a surface electromyography study. *BMC Musculoskelet Disord* 2009; 10: 78.

Fibromyalgia

Chapter 8

Endocrine theories

Introduction

Endocrine changes have been studied for a long time in determining the causation of fibromyalgia. Changes in various hormonal axes have been found in patients with fibromyalgia. This chapter will elaborate on the various endocrine theories aiming to explain the aetiology of fibromyalgia syndrome.

Neuroendocrine abnormalities

Pain physiological pathways are modulated by the autonomic nervous system and the hypothalamic-pituitary-adrenal (HPA) axis. In fibromyalgia, changes in the HPA axis are evident as described below.

The endocrine theory involving cortisol

It has been found that the levels of cortisol, a hormone released by the adrenal glands during stressful situations, are altered in patients with fibromyalgia. This suggests that changes in cortisol level could be contributing to fibromyalgia.

Stress and pain activate the neurons that secrete corticotrophin-releasing hormone (CRH), leading to adrenocorticotrophic hormone (ACTH) release and a decrease in pain symptoms. However, in patients with fibromyalgia, research has shown hyperactivity of the HPA axis. In these patients, there is a significant increase of ACTH release under CRH stimulation, with urinary free cortisol levels remaining unchanged.

Studies have demonstrated that CRH levels in the cerebrospinal fluid (CSF) are associated with sensory and affective symptoms, but not with fatigue. This strongly indicates a direct correlation between CRH levels and pain symptoms in fibromyalgia.

The endocrine theory involving other hormones

Abnormally low levels of other hormones, namely serotonin, noradrenaline and dopamine, have been found in the brain in patients with fibromyalgia. This can possibly explain the chemical imbalances that cause fibromyalgia.

Stress system plasticity at the endocrine level

Genetic and environmental factors have been proposed as possible contributors to causing changes to the central CRH neurocircuit activity and the responsiveness of the HPA axis. Adverse childhood experiences, including abuse and neglect, for example, could be a contributing factor underlying the aetiology of fibromyalgia via abnormal CRH and HPA activities.

Growth hormone in the aetiopathogenesis of fibromyalgia

Growth hormone (GH) and insulin-like growth factor I (IGF-I) are hormones required for muscle maintenance and repair. Sleep problems are known to lead to abnormal secretion of these two hormones. Low levels of GH and IGF-I have been noted in patients with fibromyalgia. GH axis disturbances, either through GH deficiency or resistance to the actions of GH, have been demonstrated in fibromyalgia. IGF-I has been used as a screening tool for investigating the GH axis in patients with fibromyalgia.

High levels of prolactin have been found in fibromyalgia. Studies have shown the prolactin level could have a good predictive value in the diagnosis of fibromyalgia.

An endorphin deficit disorder

Endocrine changes can lead to a potential hypersecretory endogenous opioid system in fibromyalgia, as indicated by elevated CSF levels of dynorphin and Met-enkephalin-Arg-Phe levels (a unique marker for pro-enkephalin). This, in turn, could result in receptor desensitisation and decreased presynaptic inhibition of substance P in the dorsal horn, causing allodynia. Case reports have described the use of low-dose naltrexone to treat fibromyalgia, based on the assumption that fibromyalgia is an endocrine/endorphin deficit disorder.

Psychological factors and the HPA axis

Scientists have put forward cogent neuroendocrine pathways that explain how psychological factors could lead to the fibromyalgia syndrome. A central abnormality of the HPA axis has been found to be associated with reduced secretion of CRH in the hypothalamus in patients with fibromyalgia. Reduced cortisol levels are consistent with features of fatigue, somnolence and widespread pain. Depression is a frequent comorbidity in patients with fibromyalgia, in support of the neuroendocrine theory underlying disease causation.

Sleep disturbances and the neuroendocrine axis

The role of sleep disturbances in the aetiopathogenesis of fibromyalgia is discussed in detail in Chapter 10. GH is mainly secreted in stages 3 and 4 of non-rapid eye movement sleep. Studies have shown that this GH secretion is disrupted in patients with fibromyalgia, thus associating sleep disturbances with the neuroendocrine theory.

The hypothalamic-pituitary-gonadal (HPG) axis

Some groups have suggested interactions between the HPA and HPG axes, thereby affecting the levels of sex hormones. Low hypothalamic gonadotropin-releasing hormone (GnRH) levels have been found in patients with fibromyalgia.

Sex hormones and fibromyalgia

Levels of serum androgens, such as dehydroepiandrosterone (DHEA) and testosterone, have been found to be markedly low in patients with fibromyalgia. Androgens are known to have anabolic effects on muscles. Further research is warranted to determine whether fibromyalgia could be caused by anti-anabolic properties of androgens or by low androgen levels.

Stress causing low oestrogen levels has been suggested as another possible cause of fibromyalgia. Early menopause has been found to be prevalent in patients with fibromyalgia. Further studies are needed to explore whether serotonin levels, together with oestrogen levels, are reduced in fibromyalgia, which, in turn, could increase the levels of substance P and thereby cause pain.

Disturbed sympathetic system activity

It has been found that the levels of plasma neuropeptide Y, a peptide that is co-localised with noradrenaline, are low in patients with fibromyalgia, suggesting a hypoactive sympathetic nervous system in fibromyalgia.

The serotonergic pathway and HPA axis

The HPA axis is under serotonergic control. Low levels of 5-hydroxytryptamine (5-HT), or serotonin, in patients with fibromyalgia lend support to the hypothesis of dysregulation of the HPA axis as a possible aetiological factor in fibromyalgia.

Cause or effect — confusion

It remains uncertain whether the endocrine changes described in this chapter are a cause or a consequence of fibromyalgia, or simply an association similar to that found in other chronic pain conditions. It is clear, however, that these neuroendocrine changes could explain the relationship between chronic stress and fibromyalgia. But here again, uncertainty prevails, as is the case with other theories for the aetiopathogenesis of fibromyalgia — these neuroendocrine changes are not seen in all patients with fibromyalgia. Even studies conducted so far do not represent the global population of patients with fibromyalgia. Furthermore, the hormonal changes present in fibromyalgia could be either primary or an effect secondary to pain associated with the condition.

Key Points

- Hyperactivity of the HPA axis, along with increased ACTH response, is seen in fibromyalgia.
- GH and IGF-I levels are low in fibromyalgia.
- The HPG axis can be affected by low androgen and oestrogen levels.
- Low serotonin levels could explain the dysregulation of the HPA axis and the pain pathway.

References

1. NHS. Causes: fibromyalgia; 2019. Available from: https://www.nhs.uk/conditions/fibromyalgia/causes/.

2. Staud R, Domingo M. Evidence for abnormal pain processing in fibromyalgia syndrome. *Pain Med* 2001; 2(3): 208-15.

3. Pillemer SR, Bradley LA, Crofford LJ, *et al.* The neuroscience and endocrinology of fibromyalgia. *Arthritis Rheum* 1997; 40(11): 1928-39.

4. McLean SA, Williams DA, Stein PK, *et al.* Cerebrospinal fluid corticotropin-releasing factor concentration is associated with pain but not fatigue symptoms in patients with fibromyalgia. *Neuropsychopharmacology* 2006; 31(12): 2776-82.

5. Cuatrecasas G, Gonzalez MJ, Alegre C, *et al.* High prevalence of growth hormone deficiency in severe fibromyalgia syndromes. *J Clin Endocrinol Metab* 2010; 95(9): 4331-7.

6. Bellato E, Marini E, Castoldi F, *et al.* Fibromyalgia syndrome: etiology, pathogenesis, diagnosis, and treatment. *Pain Res Treat* 2012; 2012: 426130.

7. Ramanathan S, Panksepp J, Johnson B. Is fibromyalgia an endocrine/endorphin deficit disorder? Is low dose naltrexone a new treatment option? *Psychosomatics* 2012; 53(6): 591-4.

8. Gupta A, Silman AJ. Psychological stress and fibromyalgia: a review of the evidence suggesting a neuroendocrine link. *Arthritis Res Ther* 2004; 6(3): 98-106.

9. Siracusa R, Di Paola RD, Cuzzocrea S, Impellizzeri D. Fibromyalgia: pathogenesis, mechanisms, diagnosis and treatment options update. *Int J Mol Sci* 2021; 22(8): 3891.

Chapter 9

Vascular theories

Introduction

In the 1990s, much research was actively focused on the various theories for the aetiopathogenesis of fibromyalgia described in earlier chapters. However, since 2010, the vascular theories have gained increasing popularity among researchers. Many studies have been conducted on peptidergic sensory innervation of microvascular shunts in the peripheries of patients with fibromyalgia.

Microvascular pathology

Cutaneous arterioles and arteriole-venule shunts (AVS) are innervated by vasoconstrictive sympathetic, as well as vasodilatory small-fibre sensory, nerve fibres. AVS were found to receive significantly increased vasodilatory sensory innervation (compared with vasoconstrictive sympathetic fibres) in fibromyalgia, as shown in various studies using skin biopsies from patients with fibromyalgia; average innervation was increased twofold in fibromyalgia, compared to controls. Furthermore, AVS were larger (and more tortuous) in patients with fibromyalgia, compared with age-matched control subjects.

Sensory fibres express α2C receptors and are increased in number in fibromyalgia, which could explain the fact that sympathetic innervation exerts an inhibitory modulation of sensory innervation. This excessive sensory innervation could be the reason behind the severe pain experienced by patients with fibromyalgia.

Blood flow dysregulation in AVS could affect thermoregulation and cause widespread pain and fatigue in fibromyalgia. Scientists have proposed that this mechanism could explain why serotonin-noradrenaline reuptake inhibitors (SNRIs) have beneficial effects in fibromyalgia.

Excessive peptidergic sensory innervation

Small-fibre sensory innervation could play a key role in widespread dysaesthesia. All sensory nerve fibres innervating the cutaneous vasculature contain substance P and calcitonin gene-related peptide (CGRP), both of which are potent vasodilators implicated as causative factors in fibromyalgia (see Chapter 6).

Immunochemical studies of normal muscle biopsies have shown different types of innervation of AVS, including: peptidergic C and Aδ fibres, non-peptidergic Aδ fibres and noradrenergic sympathetic fibres. In fibromyalgia, there is increased CGRP-expressing nerve fibres, mostly peptidergic C-fibres, and a significant reduction in sympathetic innervation.

These peptidergic C-fibres could be directly associated with increased expression of transient receptor potential vanilloid 1 (TRPV-1) receptors, which, in turn, could explain the effectiveness of capsaicin in fibromyalgia.

AVS dysregulation and muscle ischaemia

AVS is involved in thermoregulation during exercise or physical activity. Due to increased innervation of AVS in patients with fibromyalgia, it is possible that blood flow is re-routed to superficial skin, leading to insufficient blood flow and consequently ischaemia in deep skeletal muscles, thereby causing widespread pain and fatigue.

Autonomic dysregulation in fibromyalgia

Fibromyalgia is considered to be a sympathetically mediated neuropathic pain syndrome. While sympathetic mediators, such as noradrenaline, were previously studied in relation to exercise in the context of fibromyalgia, recent studies have used heart rate variability analysis and tilt table tests in patients with fibromyalgia. There is wide agreement among scientists on a deficient sympathetic response to different types of stressors in fibromyalgia. This dysautonomia in fibromyalgia is characterised as a persistently hyperactive sympathetic system that is hyporeactive to stress.

Furthermore, studies have found a correlation between heart rate variabilities and sleep disturbances recorded on polysomnography. Excessive arousal/awakening episodes have been observed, accompanied by a preceding sympathetic surge, in patients with fibromyalgia.

Catechol-O-methyltransferase and fibromyalgia

Catechol-O-methyltransferase (COMT) is the main enzyme involved in catecholamine catabolism. Genomic studies have examined COMT defects in patients with fibromyalgia, and found that in women, failure to degrade catecholamines effectively is associated with a higher risk of developing fibromyalgia. Genetic polymorphism studies showed that the LL and LH genotypes are commoner in fibromyalgia than in controls. Another study showed that the Met/Met genotype is associated with greater severity of fibromyalgia symptoms.

Key Points

- Excessive innervation of AVS can cause blood flow dysregulation in fibromyalgia, resulting in widespread pain and fatigue.
- Dysautonomia with a persistently hyperactive sympathetic nervous system that is hyporeactive to stress has been proposed as an underlying causative mechanism in fibromyalgia.
- Research is being conducted to examine COMT polymorphism in relation to the aetiopathogenesis of fibromyalgia.

References

1. Albrecht PJ, Hou Q, Argoff CE, et al. Excessive peptidergic sensory innervation of cutaneous arteriole-venule shunts (AVS) in the palmar glabrous skin of fibromyalgia patients: implications for widespread deep tissue pain and fatigue. Pain Med 2013; 14(6): 895-915.

2. Martinez-Lavin M. Biology and therapy of fibromyalgia. Stress, the stress response system, and fibromyalgia. Arthritis Res Ther 2007; 9(4): 216.

3. Kooh M, Martínez-Lavín M, Meza S, et al. Simultaneous heart rate variability and polysomnographic analyses in fibromyalgia. Clin Exp Rheumatol 2003; 21(4): 529-30.

4. Gürsoy S, Erdal E, Herken H, et al. Significance of catechol-O-methyltransferase gene polymorphism in fibromyalgia syndrome. Rheumatol Int 2003; 23(3): 104-7.

5. Garcia-Fructuoso FJ, Lao-Villadoniga JI, Beyer K, et al. Relationship between COMT gene genotypes and severity of fibromyalgia. Rheumatol Clin 2006; 2: 168-72.

Chapter 10

Other aetiological theories

Introduction

None of the proposed theories so far can fully account for the causation of fibromyalgia. However, it is clear that clinically, whatever the aetiopathology, central sensitisation leads to chronicity and persistence of widespread pain and fatigue in fibromyalgia. This chapter will detail the other theories proposed in an attempt to explain the aetiopathogenesis of fibromyalgia.

The stress theory

Stressful events have often been considered as the trigger for fibromyalgia. These can include physical stress, such as injury, viral infection and surgery, or emotional stress, such as relationship breakdown, being in an abusive relationship and trauma from past abuse or violence or from death of a loved one. Stress as a cause of fibromyalgia has been debated as it is not always possible to find a stressful trigger in all patients suffering from the condition.

The infection theory

Various viral infections, including Epstein-Barr virus, human immunodeficiency virus (HIV), parvovirus B19 (fifth disease), coxsackievirus and viral hepatitis, have been proposed as causative factors leading to fibromyalgia.

Studies showed that 29% of patients with HIV met the diagnostic criteria for fibromyalgia. In a study of patients with chronic hepatitis C, it was found that 53% had diffuse musculoskeletal pain and 10% fulfilled the diagnostic criteria for fibromyalgia. Another similar study of hepatitis C patients showed that 16% of infected patients had fibromyalgia.

Lyme disease (a bacterial disease transmitted by ticks) has been associated with fibromyalgia, based on many patient reports suffering from both conditions, although an actual causal link between the two remains to be proven. A study of 800 patients with possible Lyme disease reported that 77 of these patients had fibromyalgia with clinical features of chronic muscle pain, fatigue and neuropsychological symptoms. The authors noted that the fibromyalgia symptoms did not improve with repeated courses of antibiotics used to treat Lyme disease.

Theories implicating infection as a cause

Two different theories have been proposed, implicating infection as a cause of fibromyalgia:

1. An infectious agent gains entry into tissues such as the nervous system or joints, and triggers pain and fatigue. However, microbiological studies have failed to demonstrate this is the case, and antibiotics and antivirals have failed to resolve these fibromyalgia-related symptoms. Furthermore, this theory does not explain why fibromyalgia symptoms persist, even after an infection has subsided or been treated successfully.
2. Rather than directly causally associated with fibromyalgia, infection can act as a trigger and promote a maladaptive behaviour pattern that secondarily leads to fibromyalgia. This 'psychosocial' model emphasises a patient's adaptation to stressful events.

The immunological theory

It has been proposed that the brain dynamically modulates the immune system, while the reverse is also true. The immune system-brain communication pathway can trigger a constellation of central nervous system-mediated changes called 'sickness responses'.

It is thought that these responses are due to the immune response stimulating the production and activation of glial cells that, in turn, release proinflammatory cytokines. These will eventually lead to enhanced pain sensitivity.

Activation of immune-mediated glial cell changes can occur at various levels, including the peripheral nerves, dorsal root ganglia, spinal cord and higher centres of the brain.

Among the proinflammatory cytokines, interleukin-1 is expressed by glial cells in the central nervous system and released rapidly by tumour necrosis factor (TNF) alpha-converting enzyme (TACE). TNF alpha is expressed on the extracellular surface of glial cells and activated upon release by TACE.

The above-mentioned 'sickness responses' can be amplified, reaching painful states, with damage to nerve fibres, which results in neuropathic responses. Dysregulation of the neural circuitry causing these neuropathic responses occurs via various mechanisms.

The psychosocial theory

Central sensitisation is well established as the main cause for persistence of pain in fibromyalgia. However, this is not a unitary phenomenon. There is a link between central, peripheral, and psychosocial sensitisation. Cognitive-emotional sensitisation has been proposed as a causative factor for increased perception of pain in fibromyalgia.

The trauma theory

Many studies have reported trauma as a predisposing factor for fibromyalgia. A trauma study from Israel showed that there is an increased rate of fibromyalgia among patients with cervical spine injury (21.6%), compared with those with other injuries (1.7%). The same study reports that fibromyalgia is 13 times more common following neck injury than following lower extremity injury.

The 'reactive' fibromyalgia theory

This theory hypothesises that a precipitating factor, such as illness or trauma, at the onset of fibromyalgia causes worsening of symptoms, leading to disability and loss of employment. 'Reactive' patients with fibromyalgia were found to have significantly reduced physical activity.

A 4-year Canadian study of patients with fibromyalgia found that 23% of patients had a specific event prior to the onset of illness such as trauma, surgery or a medical illness. The study found that those who had 'reactive' fibromyalgia had significant disability and reduced physical activity.

Research has found that 60% of patients with fibromyalgia had a precipitating factor — physical trauma 33%, illness or infection 18%, and emotional trauma 14%.

The sleep theories

It has been proposed that disturbed sleep patterns may be a cause for fibromyalgia, rather than a symptom. It is evident among patients with fibromyalgia that the majority suffer from sleep problems that lead to extreme fatigue. Poor-quality sleep is directly correlated with pain and other symptoms of fibromyalgia. See Chapter 59 for more details.

Disordered sleep physiology is linked to non-restorative sleep, fatigue, diffuse widespread pain and cognitive behavioural symptoms in patients with fibromyalgia.

Fibromyalgia is associated with poor-quality sleep and frequent awakening, which has been suggested to be due to changes in slow-wave sleep with changes at the hypothalamic level. Cytokines such as interleukin-1 (IL-1) and TNF alpha are considered to be humoral agents involved in sleep regulation. Animal studies have shown that these cytokines lead to increased intensity and duration of non-rapid eye movement (non-REM) sleep.

Slow-wave sleep also controls the release of growth hormone. In fibromyalgia, sleep fragmentation causing arousal and awakening can inhibit growth hormone secretion.

Animal studies have shown an association between sleep deprivation and immunosuppression. Prolonged duration of sleep deprivation has also been found to lead to a cachectic-like state in animals.

Polysomnography has shown specific electroencephalography (EEG) changes, including alpha wave intrusion in deep-sleep stages. However, these are non-specific and are also seen in other chronic pain states and depression.

Circadian rhythm and neuroendocrine function

The intrinsic circadian rhythm is generated by the hypothalamus. This circadian rhythm, however, is affected by environmental periodicities, especially the light-dark cycle.

The human givens theory

The human givens approach is applied to a variety of conditions, including fibromyalgia. It is based on the fact that when essential emotional needs are met and an individual's innate mental resources are used correctly, that the individual will be emotionally and mentally healthy. Imbalances in these innate resources can cause fibromyalgia, as well as other painful and psychological conditions.

Sleep is important for proper functioning. The human givens approach proposes that a dreaming brain preserves the integrity of an individual's genetic inheritance every night by metaphorically defusing expectations held in the autonomic arousal system that were not acted upon before.

The genetic theories

It is possible that science has not yet properly established a proper genetic link in fibromyalgia. It has been observed that some patients are more prone than others to developing the disease and the reasons for this is not clear. This has led some groups to hypothesise that genetic causes could trigger the condition in some patients, and not in others.

Fibromyalgia has been found to run in families, suggesting genetic mutations could be responsible for disease susceptibility. A person is at high risk of developing fibromyalgia if their parent or sibling also has the condition. It is not passed directly from parents to children, but appears to cluster within families. DNA studies of family members with fibromyalgia have shown a number of genes that could explain their susceptibility of developing the disease. These genes have also been found to be associated with depression and anxiety, thus proving a link between these symptoms and fibromyalgia.

One common genetic mutation seen in patients with fibromyalgia is the 'S' (short) allele single nucleotide polymorphism in the serotonin transporter gene.

A study using genome-wide linkage analysis with 342 microsatellite markers showed that in 116 families studied, the estimated sibling recurrence risk ratio is 13.6. The authors found that the microsatellite markers D17S2196 and D17S1294 on chromosome 17p11.2-q11.2 were suggestive of fibromyalgia. This study reinforces the genetic predisposition theory. The serotonin transporter gene (SLC64A4) and the transient receptor potential vanilloid type 2 (TRPV-2) gene are considered as the main genes conferring susceptibility to fibromyalgia.

The Chiari malformation theory

Studies have suggested a link between Chiari malformation and fibromyalgia. Crowding within the posterior cranial fossa has been associated with chronic pain and fatigue. However, these are not seen in all patients with fibromyalgia. Studies on the prevalence of Chiari malformation and cervical stenosis in patients with fibromyalgia have not found supportive evidence for this association.

The free radical theory

It has been proposed that patients with fibromyalgia produce higher levels of harmful free radicals, with reduced antioxidant capacity, thus contributing to oxidative stress. This was confirmed by a study of markers of free radical damage in 85 female patients. The central nervous system is more susceptible to damage from reactive oxygen species as it has a higher lipid content.

Triggering event and fibromyalgia

As mentioned above, many people have proposed theories associating a triggering event or reaction with fibromyalgia syndrome. A 4-year retrospective study of medical records of patients with fibromyalgia from Quebec, Canada, showed that 23% of patients had trauma, surgery or a medical illness before the onset of fibromyalgia (which the authors termed as 'reactive fibromyalgia'). The same study showed that these patients with reactive fibromyalgia were more disabled than those with primary fibromyalgia (who had no trigger or precipitating cause), with loss of employment in 70%, disability compensation in 34% and reduced physical activity in 45%. The authors concluded that developing fibromyalgia following a precipitating event can lead to a prolonged and disabling pain syndrome, with considerable social and economical implications.

Key Points

- Many theories have been proposed in an attempt to explain the aetiopathogenesis of fibromyalgia.
- Stress, infection and trauma can be triggering or precipitating factors that cause fibromyalgia.
- Sleep problems are commonly associated with fibromyalgia and this association is being studied widely.

References

1. NHS. Causes: fibromyalgia; 2019. Available from: https://www.nhs.uk/conditions/fibromyalgia/causes/.

2. Staud R, Domingo MA. Evidence of abnormal pain processing in fibromyalgia syndrome. *Pain Med* 2001; 2(3): 208-15.

3. Buskila D, Gladman DD, Langevitz P, *et al.* Fibromyalgia in human immunodeficiency virus infection. *J Rheumatol* 1990; 17(9): 1202-6.

4. Rivera J, de Diego A, Trinchet M, García Monforte A. Fibromyalgia-associated hepatitis C virus infection. *Br J Rheumatol* 1997; 36(9): 981-5.

5. Buskila D, Shnaider A, Neumann L, *et al.* Fibromyalgia in hepatitis C infection – another infectious disease relationship. *Arch Intern Med* 1997; 157(21): 2497-500.

6. Hsu VM, Patella SJ, Sigal LH. "Chronic Lyme disease" as the incorrect diagnosis in patients with fibromyalgia. *Arthritis Rheum* 1993; 36(11): 1493-500.

7. Goldenberg DL. Do infections trigger fibromyalgia? *Arthritis Rheum* 1993; 36(11): 1489-92.

8. Buskila D, Neumann L, Vaisberg G, *et al.* Increased rates of fibromyalgia following cervical spine injury. A controlled study of 161 cases of traumatic injury. *Arthritis Rheum* 1997; 40(3): 446-52.

9. Overmier JB. Sensitization, conditioning, and learning: can they help us understand somatization and disability? *Scand J Psychol* 2002; 43(2): 105-12.

10. Siracusa R, Di Paola RD, Cuzzocrea S, Impellizzeri D. Fibromyalgia: pathogenesis, mechanisms, diagnosis and treatment options update. *Int J Mol Sci* 2021; 22(8): 3891.

11. Greenfield S, Fitzcharles MA, Esdaile JM. Reactive fibromyalgia syndrome. *Arthritis Rheum* 1992; 35(6): 678-81.

12. Watkins LR, Maier SF. Immune regulation of central nervous system functions: from sickness responses to pathological pain. *J Intern Med* 2005; 257(2): 139-55.

13. Pillemer SR, Bradley LA, Crofford LJ, *et al.* The neuroscience and endocrinology of fibromyalgia. *Arthritis Rheum* 1997; 40(11): 1928-39.

14. Human Givens Institute. What are the 'human givens'? Available from: https://www.hgi.org.uk/human-givens/introduction/what-are-human-givens.

15. Mayo Clinic. Fibromyalgia. Available from: https://www.mayoclinic.org/diseases-conditions/fibromyalgia/symptoms-causes/syc-20354780.

16. Mayo Clinic. Is fibromyalgia hereditary?; 2020. Available from: https://www.mayoclinic.org/diseases-conditions/fibromyalgia/expert-answers/is-fibromyalgia-hereditary/faq-20058091.

17. Bellato E, Marini E, Castoldi F, *et al.* Fibromyalgia syndrome: etiology, pathogenesis, diagnosis, and treatment. *Pain Res Treat* 2012; 2012: 426130.

18. Arnold LM, Fan J, Russell IJ, *et al.* The fibromyalgia family study: a genome-wide linkage scan study. *Arthritis Rheum* 2013; 65(4): 1122-8.

19. Bradley LA, Alarcón GS. Is Chiari malformation associated with increased levels of substance P and clinical symptoms in persons with fibromyalgia? *Arthritis Rheum* 1999; 42(12): 2731-2.

20. Clauw DJ, Bennett RM, Petzke F, *et al.* Prevalence of Chiari malformation and cervical stenosis in fibromyalgia. *Arthritis Rheum* 2000; 43: S173.

21. Bagis S, Tamer L, Sahin G, *et al.* Free radicals and antioxidants in primary fibromyalgia: an oxidative stress disorder? *Rheumatol Int* 2005; 25(3): 188-90.

Fibromyalgia

Chapter 11

Risk factors for fibromyalgia

Introduction

A recent review of 37 different research papers on fibromyalgia showed that the risk factors for fibromyalgia included childhood trauma, female sex, increased age, smoking, obesity and pre-existing medical disorders. The strongest associations were seen with sleep disorders, headaches, depression and illness.

Age

Fibromyalgia can affect any age and can also affect children. It is commonly diagnosed in middle-aged individuals and the risk increases with age.

Sex

Women are at twice the risk of presenting with fibromyalgia compared with men. Some studies have even shown up to a four times higher incidence of fibromyalgia in women.

Associated medical conditions

Associated comorbid conditions present with a higher risk of showing symptoms of fibromyalgia. Lupus and rheumatoid arthritis are associated with a greater risk of secondary fibromyalgia.

Psychosocial risk factors

Psychiatric conditions and poor coping skills can predispose individuals to fibromyalgia.

Patients with fibromyalgia who have depression report more somatic symptoms and have severe pain scores.

Women with a history of childhood sexual abuse have more somatic symptoms in fibromyalgia. This history correlates with the number of symptoms and their severity.

Role of violence in women

A Spanish comparative study of 574 participants showed that women who were unemployed were at a greater risk than women in employment. Abuse was more prevalent in the fibromyalgia group than in the control group; however, the differences were not statistically significant. This study showed that level of education was inversely proportional to the probability of developing fibromyalgia.

Childhood trauma

In a study of women with fibromyalgia, a history of trauma in childhood was related to markedly low levels of cortisol at the time of first awakening from sleep. This substantiated the neuroendocrine pathway in the causation of the disease. In this study, sexual abuse in childhood was the second predictor of cortisol level diurnal changes.

Another comparative study of patients with fibromyalgia with somatoform pain disorders and a control group described that the fibromyalgia patient group documented the highest score for childhood adversities. In this study, in addition to sexual and physical maltreatment, patients with fibromyalgia reported having poor emotional relationships with both parents.

Socioeconomic status

Studies have shown that fibromyalgia is more common in patients of lower socioeconomic status (risk ratio of 3.6).

Obesity

A higher prevalence of obesity (40%) and overweight (30%) was seen in patients with fibromyalgia, as detailed in epidemiological studies. However, it was difficult to predict if this prevalence was a cause, an association or an effect of the disease. Various mechanisms have been proposed to explain the link between obesity and fibromyalgia. These include reduced physical activity, cognitive and sleep disturbances, psychological effects including depression, thyroid dysfunction, dysfunction of growth hormone and the IGF-1 axis, and an impaired endogenous opioid system.

Genetic risk factors

One large genotyping study showed that certain alleles were found more frequently (TAAR1, RGS4, CNR1, GRIA4) and were more common in patients with fibromyalgia. Whether these alleles could be targets for diagnosis or intervention needs to be researched in the future with studies showing reproducible results.

Risk factors for psychological distress in fibromyalgia

In patients presenting with fibromyalgia, there are predictors of higher psychological distress; these include hypervigilance, less acceptance and less perceived social support. The researchers suggested that illness cognition, pain avoidance and social support could be used as prognostic factors for predicting psychological distress in patients with fibromyalgia.

Menstrual history and fibromyalgia

Studies have estimated that patients with fibromyalgia had a significantly later menarche (odds ratio of 2.2 for later than 14 years old). The incidence of women not being pregnant was higher in the fibromyalgia group. It is difficult to conclude whether these observations are the risk factors or the effects of fibromyalgia.

Key Points

- **Fibromyalgia is more common in women, older individuals, or those diagnosed with obesity or with pre-existing medical illnesses.**
- **Childhood trauma or a past history of trauma or abuse can be associated with fibromyalgia.**
- **Fibromyalgia is associated with psychological distress; poor coping skills can lead to chronicity in these patients.**

References

1. Creed F. A review of the incidence and risk factors for fibromyalgia and chronic widespread pain in population-based studies. *Pain* 2020; 161(6): 1169-76.

2. Centers for Disease Control and Prevention. Fibromyalgia. Available from: https://www.cdc.gov/arthritis/basics/fibromyalgia.htm.

3. Staud R, Domingo MA. Evidence of abnormal pain processing in fibromyalgia syndrome. *Pain Med* 2001; 2(3): 208-15.

4.   Ruiz-Pérez I, Plazaola-Castaño J, Cáliz-Cáliz R, *et al.* Risk factors for fibromyalgia: the role of violence against women. *Clin Rheumatol* 2009; 28(7): 777-86.

5.   Weissbecker I, Floyd A, Dedert E, *et al.* Childhood trauma and diurnal cortisol disruption in fibromyalgia syndrome. *Psychoneuroendocrinology* 2006; 31(3): 312-24.

6.   Imbierowicz K, Egle UT. Childhood adversities in patients with fibromyalgia and somatoform pain disorder. *Eur J Pain* 2003; 7(2): 113-9.

7.   Schochat T, Beckmann C. Sociodemographic characteristics, risk factors and reproductive history in subjects with fibromyalgia – results of a population-based case-control study. *Z Rheumatol* 2003; 62(1): 46-59.

8.   Ursini F, Naty S, Grembiale RD. Fibromyalgia and obesity: the hidden link. *Rheumatol Int* 2011; 31(11): 1403-8.

9.   Smith SB, Maixner DW, Fillingim RB, *et al.* Large candidate gene association study reveals genetic risk factors and therapeutic targets for fibromyalgia. *Arthritis Rheum* 2012; 64(2): 584-93.

10.   van Koulil, van Lankveld W, Kraaimaat FW, *et al.* Risk factors for longer term psychological distress in well-functioning fibromyalgia patients: a prospective study into prognostic factors. *Patient Educ Couns* 2010; 80(1): 126-9.

Fibromyalgia

Section 3

Clinical examination

Fibromyalgia

Chapter 12

Patient history and gaining a rapport

Introduction

Many patients with fibromyalgia feel that they are not believed by healthcare professionals and the wider public. Given their wide spectrum of multiple symptoms, they find it difficult to explain their problems during a single consultation. Furthermore, 'brain fog' and memory problems can make their healthcare consultation challenging.

A survey of physicians and medical students who were asked to order medical diseases in a hierarchy of prestigiousness unfortunately concluded that fibromyalgia was the least or lowest prestigious disease! Even though this study was carried out more than a decade ago, the author of this book feels, with anguish, that the perceptions of healthcare professionals still hold true and need to be changed. These hierarchies can stigmatise the perception of healthcare staff towards patients with fibromyalgia.

Many doctors and healthcare professionals regard these patients as 'time consuming' and 'resource consuming'. However, if healthcare professionals can create a rapport with the patient and make them believe that they are keen to listen to their problems, this ensures the consultation is productive and successful.

Patients' experiences

One study showed that fibromyalgia evoked uneasiness in healthcare staff and placed great demand on resources in clinical practice. In these patients, there are complex interrelationships and needs between physical, psychological and social domains; these needs should be explored by clinicians to produce a successful consultation. The study concluded that taking a more holistic approach would help to manage the somatic and psychosocial symptom profile of these patients in a more effective way.

Many patients felt that the legitimacy of the diagnosis itself was questioned by many medical staff; this can lead to many patients feeling that their identity and core integrity are under question.

Inclusiveness

For a long time, the National Health Service in the UK has maintained the goal of patient inclusiveness in order to deliver a high-quality personal service. The NHS aims to ensure that public and patient voices are at the centre of shaping our healthcare services.

Preparation before the clinic

Many patients with fibromyalgia have already seen several specialists in different clinics without satisfaction. The 'revolving-door' phenomenon is used as a metaphor in which these patients go from one clinic to other, sometimes with no one taking the responsibility of engaging them in a biopsychosocial model.

Healthcare professionals should be prepared to be empathetic with the feelings of patients with fibromyalgia. We should accept their emotional expressions including frustration, anger and despair. It may be wise to say that we believe their pain (which contradicts previous opinions as 'all in your head') and evoke their confidence to obtain better rapport, which will then lead to future engagement in the various management options of the healthcare services.

The first visit

The first consultation should provide the patient with sufficient confidence that someone is listening to their problems. Active listening can be a very effective communication tool with these patients. The evaluation is not one-sided, in that the patient also evaluates the clinician and their sincere efforts to understand their pain/feelings; this can have a profound lasting impact on the outcome of the treatment.

Eye contact and body language

A good clinical consultation necessitates good communication skills; maintaining eye contact, good listening skills and showing compassion with body language are vital for patients with fibromyalgia. Showing empathy by active listening is the key to engaging in believing the patient's clinical distress from their perspective.

Both verbal and non-verbal cues should be used by the clinician to demonstrate that the patient is being actively listened to.

Repeating back what the patient says in a summarised form intermittently and regularly can help to ensure that the clinician has correctly understood their narrative, and ensures that the patient believes that we have heard their complaints.

I believe your pain

It is essential that a patient with fibromyalgia has confidence that the listening consultant believes that his/her pain is real. The clinician should constantly provide this confidence by both verbal and non-verbal cues. Verbal confirmation that the clinician believes their pain is real will secure a better rapport when helping to prepare a patient-directed self-management plan.

Giving the verbal confidence that the clinician believes the pain is real does not mean that the treatment should deviate from the biopsychosocial model. Explaining that their description of pain is believed, but at the same time detailing the scientific evidence for the biopsychosocial pathway for management strategies, will yield better success when engaging with the comprehensive treatment plan.

Asking about patients' expectations

Understanding the patient's expectations is vital to understanding their needs and creating a better rapport with the patient; this should be actively questioned by the clinician when treating patients with fibromyalgia. It might be that the expectations of the clinician and the patient differ, but it is important to understand and explain the reasons for these differences.

It will be a significant challenge if the patient expects a cure rather than management for fibromyalgia; publications have stressed the need to align patient expectations at the point of referral with what can be realistically achieved. This might be difficult in some situations, but education by the referring primary care physician, providing leaflets with adequate explanation to the patient about what can be achieved in the pain clinic before they come to the clinic, and explaining this again before the consultation might help to direct the consultation in an appropriate manner.

Asking about patients' concerns/worries

It is important to ask if the patient has any concerns or worries; each patient will have different goals and different concerns. Whilst one patient might be worried how their pain might worsen in the future, another might be concerned about their job or family. Asking for their concerns and answering these questions will immensely benefit the patient.

Calm competent approach

Sometimes patients might be anxious or frustrated; it is prudent for the healthcare professional to be calm and, at the same time, demonstrate their knowledge and skills in a competent manner. History taking is not only a skill, but is also an art, especially when dealing with patients with fibromyalgia.

Taking a detailed history

Many aspects of standard history-taking apply for fibromyalgia after considering the above empathetic approach; this chapter details the specifics needed for patients with fibromyalgia:

- Detailed history of the presenting complaint.
- Details of pain: site, onset, characteristics, radiation, associations, timing, exacerbating/relieving factors, severity (SOCRATES).
- Past medical history.
- Medications taken and those tried in the past.
- Other treatments tried and their effectiveness.
- Psychological history: how do they cope with and manage their pain; are there any catastrophising factors; how does the pain affect their mood and day-to-day life; how is their sleep affected; how is their relationship with their family affected; are there any secondary gains?
- Social history: work and workplace problems; receiving benefits or support; their social interactions, etc.
- History of allergies, smoking and alcohol intake.
- Family history.
- Summarising the history back to the patient.
- Asking the patient whether we have missed any other problems.

The steps required in history taking for fibromyalgia are outlined in ▓ Table 12.1.

Table 12.1. Steps in history taking for fibromyalgia.

	Process	Goals
1	Introduction/check if it is the right patient	Wishing and smiling to achieve a rapport
2	Seated/position as they wish	Make sure they are comfortable
3	Explain the pain clinic process/details from referral of which you are already aware	Provide a good introduction and show that you are interested to hear more narration
4	Details of present complaints	To understand the nature of the pain and other symptoms (SOCRATES)
5	Explain that you believe the patient's pain	Showing empathy and evoking confidence
6	Summarising history back to the patient	Gives confidence to the patient that you are listening actively
7	Past medical history	Details from past history
8	Medications history	Drugs that are used now and that have been tried before
9	Therapies history	Other treatments tried and whether they were effective
10	Activities of daily living	Assessing what activities are limited due to the pain
11	Asking how they feel	Assessing psychological history and how they cope with the pain
12	Sleep history	Assess how the pain affects their sleep in the night-time, whether they feel refreshed after sleep, whether they take naps in the daytime

Table 12.1 *continued*. Steps in history taking for fibromyalgia.

	Process	Goals
13	Occupational history	To understand how the pain affects their work life, their financial concerns, whether they are receiving disability benefits
14	Social history	Assess how their social life is affected due to the pain/fatigue
15	Other histories	History of smoking, alcohol, drugs; any allergies
16	Asking about patient's expectations	Will help to set the goals for the management plan and making sure they are in line with what could be achieved from the service
17	Asking about patient's worries/concerns	Aims to remove catastrophising worries and provide an explanation
18	Ask if we have missed any other problems in the medical history	To check that nothing else is missed

Standardising the biopsychosocial model in the framework

The biopsychosocial model (see Chapter 17) is the cornerstone of clinical management of patients with fibromyalgia; even at the history-taking stage, this should be the main framework and the psychosocial aspects should be given the same priority as the questions related to the physical components. Establishing a rapport during the history-taking part of the consultation should initiate the concepts of the biopsychosocial model, so that it will be easier during the final part of the consultation, when this is used as the basis for a comprehensive management plan.

Narrative medicine

Despite enormous scientific advances, clinicians find it difficult to extend empathy towards many chronic pain patients, in particular those with fibromyalgia. It needs special competence to be honest and courageously listen to the plight and the needs of these patients. Along with the medical competence that comes with training at medical/professional schools, clinicians need the ability to listen, grasp and honour the meaning of the patient narrative (their journey through the disease and their experiences). This narrative competence can enable the healthcare professional to practise their skills with empathy, reflection, professionalism and trustworthiness.

Consultation as therapy

Clinicians should determine themselves if the consultation itself could be management or therapy, or at least the initiation of these. Patients with fibromyalgia often express that they have experienced symptoms for long periods, in that they have felt that no one in the past has listened to their problems. Specialist doctors could have looked at what they could correct based on their own specialist training and might have sent these patients through a 'revolving-door' phenomenon and therefore the search for a 'magic wand' or solution would have continued for a long time. Getting the patients to be engaged in a biopsychosocial model, listening to their history and concerns, and explaining the management model that looks at taking control of pain in their own hands, these goals will themselves be the initial therapy for their condition. The doctor taking part in the consultation should bear this in mind when harnessing the power of communication skills to make a change in these patients' quality of life.

Key Points

- Listening actively and showing empathy are key to the success of communication with a patient with fibromyalgia.
- The patient should be clearly informed and convinced that the clinician believes their pain.
- It is important to ask about the patient's expectations from the consultation and their concerns/worries.
- A biopsychosocial model is the cornerstone of the management of fibromyalgia and this should be clearly detailed during the initial part of the consultation itself.

References

1. Album D, Westin S. Do diseases have a prestige hierarchy? A survey among physicians and medical students. *Soc Sci Med* 2008; 66(1): 182-8.

2. Lempp HK, Hatch SL, Carville SF, Choy EH. Patients' experiences of living with and receiving treatment for fibromyalgia syndrome: a qualitative study. *BMC Musculoskelet Disord* 2009; 10: 124.

3. Darzi A. High quality of care for all: NHS next stage review final report. Department of Health; 2008.

4. Starz T. Straightforward approach can help rheumatology health professionals engage with fibromyalgia patients. The Rheumatologist 2017. Available from: https://www.the-rheumatologist.org/article/straightforward-approach-can-help-rheumatology-health-professionals-engage-fibromyalgia-patients/?singlepage=1&theme=print-friendly.

5. Bhana N, Thompson L, Alchin J, Thompson B. Patient expectations for chronic pain management. *J Prim Health Care* 2015; 7(2): 130-6.

6. Charon R. The patient-physician relationship. Narrative medicine: a model for empathy, reflection, profession, and trust. *JAMA* 2001; 286(15): 1897-902.

Fibromyalgia

Chapter 13

Clinical features

Introduction

Widespread pain and fatigue are the most common clinical presentations of fibromyalgia syndrome, although patients also commonly present with sleep, and emotional and cognitive problems.

Clinical symptoms in fibromyalgia

Common symptoms that are reported in fibromyalgia include:

- Widespread pain all over the body.
- Fatigue.
- Stiffness all over the body.
- Unrefreshing sleep, insomnia and other sleep problems.
- Problems with thinking, memory and concentration (brain fog).
- Low mood and anxiety.

Associated symptoms

Fibromyalgia is a spectrum of functional pain disorders and can include many other painful conditions including:

- Headaches and migraines.
- Functional bowel disorder or irritable bowel disorder.

- Painful bladder syndrome.
- Pelvic pain.
- Tingling and numbness in the hands and feet in a non-dermatomal pattern.
- Temporomandibular joint syndrome with pain in the jaw and/or face.
- Low back pain or neck pain.
- Autonomic disturbances.

Widespread pain and dysaesthesia

Widespread or regional pain is due to distorted pain or sensory processing in fibromyalgia. Researchers have mentioned that fibromyalgia is probably the most important and extensively described central pain syndrome.

Patients state that the pain is present all over the body; there is no anatomical or dermatomal distribution in these patients. They feel that the pain worsens with cold weather, stress, overuse or inactivity, and poor sleep.

Widespread myalgia (muscle pain) is commonly seen in fibromyalgia; this has changed the criteria for diagnosis from trigger points in the past to a Widespread Pain Index (see Chapter 14). Nearly 40% of patients also report leg cramps. Muscle function is globally impaired and strength is reduced.

Generalised stiffness all over the body is one of the symptoms of fibromyalgia. Stiffness is worse on awakening in the morning and in the evening. Patients also feel a swollen sensation in the hands and feet.

Allodynia

Allodynia is pain due to stimulus that normally does not provoke pain. For example, a light touch sensation causing pain is termed allodynia. This is commonly seen in fibromyalgia. Patients complain that even a light touch or the feeling of clothes on their bodies can cause severe pain.

Hyperalgesia

Hyperalgesia is a heightened response to a normally painful stimuli. This response could be due to lowering of the nociceptor threshold level or a heightened response in the nociplastic pathway.

Paraesthesia

Sensations of tingling, pins and needles, or numbness are felt in 84% of patients with fibromyalgia. These symptoms could mimic a neurological disorder, but the clinician can differentiate this if there is no radicular distribution.

Fatigue

Fatigue is very common in fibromyalgia and is worse in the morning. Unless well educated in the biopsychosocial pathway, patients fear doing exercise in case this worsens their pain. The term 'fatigue' can encompass different types as listed below:

- Muscle fatigue: common and any movement causes worsening tiredness.
- Pain-related fatigue.
- Stiffness-related fatigue.
- Arousal fatigue due to inadequate sleep or poor-quality sleep (see Chapter 59).
- Motivational fatigue due to low mood.

Non-refreshing sleep

Patients complain that they feel more tired and exhausted on awakening in the morning than when they went to bed the previous night. Studies have reported an incidence of 75–90% for moderate to severe fatigue.

It has been reported that 75% of patients with fibromyalgia can have sleep problems. Poor sleep can worsen pain and this can further lead to disturbed sleep that can form a vicious cycle. Non-restorative sleep is associated with the loss of stages 3 and 4 sleep (deep stages).

Polysomnographic studies have shown that patients with fibromyalgia have poorer sleep quality than a control group of patients. The studies showed that the fibromyalgia group had more periods of awakenings, a higher arousal index, greater Apnoea-Hypopnea Index and less N1 sleep. One of the studies concluded that sleep studies could distinguish patients with fibromyalgia with a 78.5% accuracy compared with healthy controls.

Brain fog/cognitive dysfunction

Fibro-fog or brain fog is the common term used to describe the related neurocognitive problems. An inability to concentrate, memory problems, reduced performance, cognitive overload and attention problems are a few of the symptoms that are mentioned by patients with fibromyalgia. These problems can lead to difficulties in organising tasks and delays in responding to questions.

Research using functional magnetic resonance imaging (fMRI) scans has shown that the memory deficit in fibromyalgia is due to differences in neural activation of the frontoparietal memory network; this could be due to both the pain itself and to mood changes (depression and anxiety). Patients with fibromyalgia showed an ageing effect that required an increased use of cognitive resources to maintain comparable levels of performance as their same-aged controls.

Neurocognitive assessment tests have shown significant incidences of distraction in patients with fibromyalgia. The auditory consonant trigram test was the most sensitive; patients with fibromyalgia lost information at a 58% rate following a 9-second distraction. This loss was disproportionate to the loss due to memory problems.

Anxiety and depression

A meta-analysis of research studies concluded that patients with fibromyalgia had a higher prevalence of depression and anxiety, with reports of 20–80% and 13–64%, respectively. It has been shown that psychological distress is more frequent and severe in patients with fibromyalgia than in controls with widespread pain of other origin.

Common symptoms on long-term follow-up

An intensive longitudinal study followed up in patients for 90 days found that unrefreshing sleep, fatigue and pain were the most intense symptoms, followed by memory problems, stress, anxiety and depression.

Clinical features and gender

A comparative study between men and women with fibromyalgia concluded that male patients showed fewer symptoms and had fewer tender points. Other symptoms such as fatigue and irritable bowel also occurred less in men.

Another study also concluded that clinical features were similar in both sexes but that female patients were subjected to a longer duration of chronic widespread pain and a higher tender point count.

Patient preference on managing clinical features

A United States patient preference study of 788 confirmed patients with fibromyalgia categorised symptoms into six clusters: pain, fatigue, domestic (effect on family), impairment (daily tasks, driving), affective (mood-related) and social clusters. Of these, the pain cluster was ranked as globally important by 54% of patients that needed intervention, followed by fatigue in 28% of patients.

Key Points

- Widespread pain and fatigue are the commonest symptoms of fibromyalgia.
- Cognitive problems or brain fog (fibro-fog) are mentioned by many patients.
- Non-refreshing or poor-quality sleep is seen in 75% of patients with fibromyalgia.
- Anxiety and depression are common in fibromyalgia.

References

1. Cassisi G, Sarzi-Puttini P, Casale R, *et al*. Pain in fibromyalgia and related conditions. *Reumatismo* 2014; 66(1): 72-86.

2. Cassisi G, Sarzi-Puttini P, Alciati A, *et al*. Symptoms and signs in fibromyalgia syndrome. *Reumatismo* 2008; 60 Suppl 1: 15-24.

3. Çetin B, Sünbül EA, Toktaş H, *et al*. Comparison of sleep structure in patients with fibromyalgia and healthy controls. *Sleep Breath* 2020; 24(4): 1591-8.

4. Seo J, Kim SH, Kim YT, *et al*. Working memory impairment in fibromyalgia patients associated with altered frontoparietal memory network. *PLoS ONE* 2012; 7(6): e37808.

5. Leavitt F, Katz RS. Distraction as a key determinant of impaired memory in patients with fibromyalgia. *J Rheumatol* 2006; 33(1): 127-32.

6. Fietta P, Fietta P, Manganelli P. Fibromyalgia and psychiatric disorders. *Acta Biomed* 2007; 78(2): 88-95.

7. Toussaint L, Vincent A, McAllister SJ, Whipple M. Intra- and inter-patient symptom variability in fibromyalgia: results of a 90-day assessment. *Musculoskelet Care* 2015; 13(2): 93-100.

8. Yunus MB, Inanici F, Aldag JC, Mangold RF. Fibromyalgia in men: comparison of clinical features with women. *J Rheumatol* 2000; 27(2): 485-90.

9. Häuser W, Kühn-Becker H, von Wilmoswky HV, *et al*. Demographic and clinical features of patients with fibromyalgia syndrome of different settings: a gender comparison. *Gend Med* 2011; 8(2): 116-25.

10. Bennett RM, Russell J, Cappelleri JC, *et al*. Identification of symptom and functional domains that fibromyalgia patients would like to see improved: a cluster analysis. *BMC Musculoskelet Disord* 2010; 11: 134.

Chapter 14

Criteria for fibromyalgia diagnosis

Introduction

It is important to understand the clinical criteria for diagnosis of fibromyalgia syndrome as it lacks specific laboratory, physical or pathological findings. The criteria for diagnosis of fibromyalgia have evolved significantly over the last few decades. Starting from identifying trigger points in the 1990s to the evaluation of widespread pain, and including symptom severity, the way that we now diagnose fibromyalgia has changed. This chapter will detail the present guidelines for diagnosis and then summarise the past guidelines for historic importance.

Basic pre-requisite for diagnosis

Fibromyalgia is a diagnosis of exclusion. Any diagnostic criteria will specify this clearly at the outset. The patient should not have a disorder that would otherwise explain the pain. This makes the diagnostic criteria complex in that the clinician should have the skills and expertise to rule out other complex conditions that could cause pain. A basic set of investigations to rule out inflammatory, endocrine and other causes of pain is essential before moving onto the diagnostic criteria of fibromyalgia.

Symptoms should be chronic; they should have lasted at a similar level for at least 3 months.

American College of Rheumatology diagnostic criteria for fibromyalgia 2010

In May 2010, the American College of Rheumatology (ACR) (Wolfe and colleagues) set specific criteria for the diagnosis of fibromyalgia; this was completely different from the criteria of trigger points that existed before 2010.

ACR 2010 criteria measure two domains:

- Widespread Pain Index (WPI)(■ Figure 14.1).
- Symptom Severity (SS) scale score.

The Widespread Pain Index (WPI) is the number of areas in which pain was felt in the previous week. This is scored between 0 and 19, based on 19 areas. These 19 areas include:

- Neck, upper back, lower back.
- Left jaw, right jaw, chest, abdomen.
- Left shoulder girdle, right shoulder girdle, left upper arm, left lower arm, right upper arm, right lower arm.
- Left hip, right hip, left upper leg, left lower leg, right upper leg, right lower leg.

The Symptom Severity (SS) scale score looks at four symptom domains and puts these into four grades (0 to 3 each); this gives a total score of 0 to 12, as below:

- Fatigue, scored 0 for no problem, 1 for mild, 2 for moderate and 3 for severe.
- Waking unrefreshed, scored 0 for no problem, 1 for mild, 2 for moderate and 3 for severe.
- Cognitive symptoms, scored 0 for no problem, 1 for mild, 2 for moderate and 3 for severe.
- Somatic symptoms, scored 0 if no symptoms, 1 if few, 2 if moderate number and 3 if great deal of symptoms.

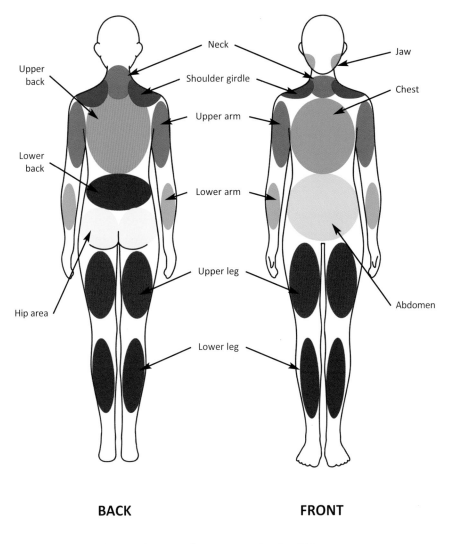

BACK FRONT

Figure 14.1. Widespread Pain Index — ACR criteria 2010.

Both these scores are added together to give the diagnostic criteria when:

- WPI ≥7 and SS ≥5; or
- WPI 3–6 and SS ≥9.

At the same time, it should fulfil the other two pre-requisite criteria mentioned at the beginning of this chapter:

- Symptoms should have been at a similar level for at least 3 months.
- The patient does not have a disorder that would otherwise explain the pain.

The Widespread Pain Index — ACR criteria 2010 — is shown in ▓ Figure 14.1.

ACR fibromyalgia classification criteria 1990

The older criteria looked at tender points (tenderness on pressure on specified areas); at least 11 of 18 specified sites were needed to diagnose fibromyalgia. Research showed that this method of diagnosis had a sensitivity of 88.4% and specificity of 81.1%. The criteria had a pre-requisite that the pain should be widespread (axial plus upper and lower segment plus left- and right-sided pain). The authors used dolorimetry and produced tender points at a pressure of a 4kg mark; this is difficult to reproduce in regular clinical practice. Fibromyalgia is a symptom-based diagnosis and these criteria had to be revised in 2010. Furthermore, these criteria did not recognise the importance of fatigue, and cognitive and somatic symptoms in the syndrome.

The trigger points in diagnosis — ACR criteria 1990 — are shown in ▓ Figure 14.2.

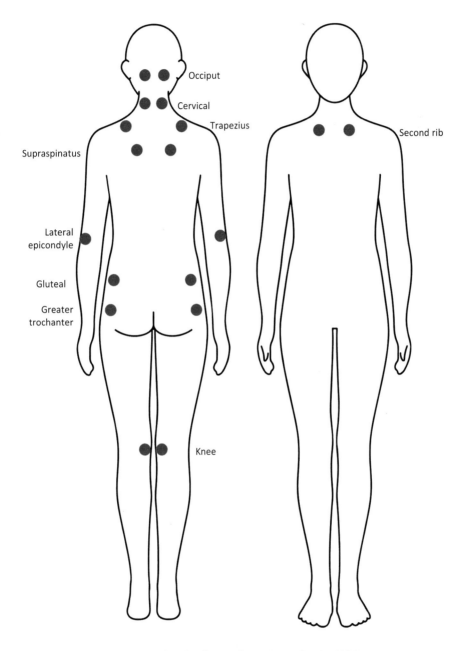

Figure 14.2. Trigger points in diagnosis — ACR criteria 1990.

Further advances in criteria

In 2011 and 2016, Wolfe and colleagues revised and modified the 2010 criteria; a polysymptomatic distress scale was used in fibromyalgia; the authors proposed this scale to facilitate its use in epidemiological or community settings. This modified the scores so that the patient could self-administer these criteria and diagnose their condition. The 2011 modified criteria looks at eliminating the physician's estimate of somatic symptoms and substituting the patient self-reported symptoms score.

In 2016, a systematic review of 2010 and 2011 criteria was published.

Future expectations in diagnostic criteria

A public-private partnership of the United States Food and Drug Administration (US FDA) and the American Pain Society (APS) formed ACTTION (Analgesic, Anaesthetic, and Addiction Clinical Trial Translations Innovations Opportunities and Networks). They formed the alternative ACTTION-APS pain taxonomy that caters for the diagnosis of a variety of chronic pain disorders, including fibromyalgia. This looks at the core diagnostic criteria, common features, common comorbidities, consequences and putative mechanisms.

The meaning of diagnosis and criteria

Whilst a diagnosis is most needed to answer a patient's questions and to legitimise their illness, the meaning of the diagnosis and the need for a biopsychosocial model is widely debated.

A patient might want a diagnosis not only to obtain treatment but also to give meaning to their illness experience. This may be uncertain for patients with fibromyalgia. A qualitative study of patients with fibromyalgia showed that the diagnosis still left them with limited meaning due to various factors: the ambiguous definition within the medical literature, the invisible nature of the illness, and the lack of an environment where these uncertainties could be openly discussed. The study concluded that patients varied in their degree of long-term acceptance of the diagnosis, in relation to the concordance they achieved between the diagnosis and their experience of the illness.

Diagnosis in clinical practice

Although we have evolved significantly from the biological concept of tender points to looking at somatic scales, the diagnostic criteria should be made easier to use by the practising busy clinician, rather than just focusing on research criteria. Most practising clinicians follow a pattern recognition scheme that is continuously updated by intrinsic and extrinsic educational neurosignature patterns. Fibromyalgia is one of the easiest, as well as one of the most difficult conditions, to diagnose as the basic pre-requisite needed is to exclude other causes of the symptoms.

Key Points

- Fibromyalgia is diagnosed clinically, with the pre-requisites of excluding other causes and symptoms need to be chronic.
- The ACR 2010 criteria focus on the WPI and the Symptom Severity score scale.
- Previous criteria of tender points are not specific for symptoms in fibromyalgia.

References

1. Wolfe F, Clauw DJ, Fitzcharles MA, *et al.* The American College of Rheumatology preliminary diagnostic criteria for fibromyalgia and measurement of symptoms severity. *Arthritis Care Res* 2010; 62(5): 600-10.

2. Wolfe F, Smythe HA, Yunus MB, *et al.* The American College of Rheumatology 1990 criteria for the classification of fibromyalgia. Report of the multicenter criteria committee. *Arthritis Rheum* 1990; 33(2): 160-72.

3. Galvez-Sánchez CM, Reyes del Paso GA. Diagnostic criteria for fibromyalgia: critical review and future perspectives. *J Clin Med* 2020; 9(4): 1219.

4. Arnold LM, Bennett RM, Crofford LJ, *et al*. AAPT diagnostic criteria for fibromyalgia. *J Pain* 2019; 20(6): 611-28.

5. Madden S, Sim J. Creating meaning in fibromyalgia syndrome. *Soc Sci Med* 2006; 63(11): 2962-73.

Chapter 15

Investigations

Introduction

Fibromyalgia is a diagnosis of exclusion. Although all pain clinics engage with these patients in a biopsychosocial model for chronic condition management, it is the duty of the primary care clinician to rule out other causes before referring patients to the pain management centres. Whilst pain and fatigue could be due to numerous causes, it is wise to order only the necessary investigations based on the presentation. The most important role of the referring physician is to rule out sinister red flags before referring patients to the management pathway.

A detailed clinical examination can help the clinician to rule out other causes and focus on the needed investigations if appropriate.

Patient reassurance versus diagnostic uncertainty

Whilst it is important to reassure patients that all sinister or treatable causes have been ruled out, many patients with fibromyalgia present with medically unexplainable symptoms. A Dutch qualitative study showed that the decision to request laboratory testing was the result of complex interactions of considerations that are often conflicting. Although complying with the perceived needs of the patient for reassurance through testing, and this approach being seen as an easy, cost-effective and time-effective strategy, the ethics and long-term management of this approach could be questioned. Furthermore, this approach could lead to the 'revolving-door' phenomenon, in which the patient could go to various specialists who are all eager to find the 'one test' that has been missed. It is prudent to order investigations based on clinical presentations, with the aim of ruling out treatable or sinister causes, with an adequate explanation to the patient and the agreement to engage in a biopsychosocial model once the tests are completed and other causes are ruled out.

Yield of the investigation

An Australian general practitioner audit showed that 64.2% of patients presenting with fatigue were investigated with pathology tests. This study is more than a decade old and the numbers could now be significantly higher.

Another Australian primary care research study showed that 53% of patients presenting with fatigue were investigated using at least one pathology test. However, only 3% were given a significant clinical diagnosis based on an abnormal pathology test. Other scientific articles have quoted a yield rate of 5–9% in cases of fatigue.

Investigations and their objectives

Investigations should be ordered only if there is a clear objective related to the diagnosis by the clinician. The list outlined in ▦ Table 15.1 includes investigations and their objectives; however, it has to be clear that not all investigations are needed for any patient presenting with fibromyalgia and the tests should only be ordered based on the need and clinical presentation.

Table 15.1. Investigations and their objectives.

Common tests	What to look for
Full blood count	Persistent inflammatory causes, white blood cell disorders (infection, lymphopenia, lymphocytosis) and signs of infection; anaemia, polycythaemia and platelet disorders
C-reactive protein (CRP), erythrocyte sedimentation rate (ESR)	To rule out other inflammatory causes
Thyroid function tests	Causes for fatigue, other endocrine causes
Renal function tests (urea and electrolytes)	Renal disorders, electrolyte abnormalities causing fatigue, muscle damage
Liver function tests	Liver damage, metabolic causes
Fasting blood sugar, HbA1c	Diabetes
Urine dipstick test	Renal infection, inflammation or tumours
Rheumatological tests	To rule out rheumatological conditions
Vitamin D levels	Deficiency can commonly present with similar symptoms
Serum ferritin	Anaemia or other blood disorders
Creatine kinase	To rule out muscle problems
Bone biochemistry, myeloma screen	In older people to rule out bone-related causes
Vitamin B12 and folate levels	Deficiency can present with similar symptoms

Red flags or sinister causes

It is important that the clinician rules out all treatable causes as well as sinister red flag causes, which could include those listed below (■ Table 15.2) in cases with a similar clinical picture to fibromyalgia.

Table 15.2. Other red flag causes in cases with a similar clinical picture to fibromyalgia.

Clinical presentation	What to look for
Weight loss	Malignancy, infection or inflammation, diabetes, endocrine causes
Blood loss	Anaemia, gastric/bowel problems
Fatigue	Anaemia, diabetes, renal problems, cardiac causes, malignancy, autoimmune diseases
Shortness of breath	Anaemia, cardiac causes, respiratory causes
Liver problems	Liver damage, metabolic causes
Weakness of limbs	Spinal cord problems, neurological causes, rheumatological causes

Other investigations

In cases of localised symptoms in fibromyalgia, a clinician might request an X-ray or magnetic resonance imaging (MRI) scan but there should be an appropriate indication with action that could be taken if the suspicion is confirmed. These other investigations are carried out with the objective of ruling out other causes of fibromyalgia.

Key Points

- Fibromyalgia is a clinical diagnosis, based on the exclusion of other causes.
- The yield of tests done is very low; tests should be performed with a focus on presenting symptoms and needs, for which the suspected test abnormalities could be corrected.
- Full blood count, CRP/ESR, urea/electrolytes, thyroid function and blood sugar levels are commonly performed to complement the clinical features of fibromyalgia.
- Investigations can rule out treatable or sinister causes.

References

1. van der Weijden T, van Bokhoven MA, Dinant GJ, et al. Understanding laboratory testing in diagnostic uncertainty: a qualitative study in general practice. Br J Gen Pract 2002; 52(485): 974-80.

2. Wilson J, Morgan S, Magin PJ, van Driel ML. Fatigue – a rational approach to investigation. Aust Fam Physician 2014; 43(7): 457-61.

3. Gialamas A, Beilby JJ, Pratt NL, et al. Investigating tiredness in Australian general practice. Do pathology tests help in diagnosis? Aust Fam Physician 2003; 32(8): 663-6.

Chapter 16

Differential diagnoses

Introduction

Fibromyalgia needs pre-requisite criteria to have all other causes ruled out; expert knowledge of differential diagnoses is vital before a diagnosis and engaging the patient in a biopsychosocial model.

Myofascial differential diagnoses

Myofascial pain syndrome is characterised by localised tender areas in muscles (e.g. trapezius muscle pain), whereas pain is widespread in fibromyalgia. Usually, there are no systemic manifestations in myofascial pain syndrome.

Electrolyte imbalance-related muscle pain can present with a similar picture to fibromyalgia and could be excluded by simple routine blood tests. Hypokalaemia and hypomagnesaemia can present with weakness in hospitalised patients. Profound hypothermia can lead to muscle damage with high creatine kinase levels, but the presentation will be acute with a corroborating history.

Myositis and myopathies of various causes need to be ruled out. These can be congenital, infective, inflammatory, metabolic or drug-induced in aetiology.

Fatigue-related differential diagnoses

Chronic fatigue syndrome or myalgic encephalomyelitis presents with a similar clinical picture to fibromyalgia and is often difficult to differentiate; however, fatigue is more prominent in these conditions than pain. Furthermore, there is an ongoing subclinical inflammatory process in chronic fatigue that can be evident as a low-grade fever, lymph node enlargement, etc.

Neurological differential diagnoses

Sinister conditions such as multiple sclerosis and neurological disorders need to be ruled out; a significant history and clinical presentation will differentiate these conditions clearly from fibromyalgia. Further investigations might be needed in complex clinical presentations.

Disorders such as parkinsonism, peripheral neuropathies, spinal stenosis with myelopathy and myotonic dystrophy can present with similar widespread weakness and need to be ruled out.

Endocrine differential diagnoses

Hypothyroidism commonly presents with a confounding clinical picture to fibromyalgia; thyroid function tests can rule out this cause. Hypothyroidism can cause profound muscle weakness and fatigue.

Parathyroid disorders, autoimmune thyroiditis, growth hormone disorders, vitamin D or calcium deficiency can present with similar clinical features.

Rheumatological differential diagnoses

Secondary fibromyalgia can occur with common rheumatological diseases such as rheumatoid arthritis and systemic lupus erythematosus. However, rheumatological diseases need to be ruled out by common blood tests and anti-nuclear antibody tests.

Joint swelling is a characteristic of rheumatological diseases, but sometimes this may be less prominent, especially in the early stages. Conditions such as rheumatoid arthritis, systemic lupus erythematosus, Sjögren's syndrome, spondyloarthritis, psoriatic arthropathy, and mixed connective tissue diseases need to be ruled out, as they can present with a similar picture to fibromyalgia.

Polymyalgia rheumatica has a similar presentation to fibromyalgia; whilst polymyalgia is believed to be an inflammatory disease with a probable autoimmune cause, fibromyalgia differs with an abnormal sensory processing aetiology. Polymyalgia usually resolves after a few years, whereas fibromyalgia is a chronic disease.

Psychiatric/psychological differential diagnoses

Anxiety disorders, somatoform pain disorders, depression, or post-traumatic stress disorder can all present with widespread pain, but a clear history and clinical features can differentiate these from fibromyalgia. As fibromyalgia and other chronic pain conditions can co-exist, it is important to exclude any psychiatric causes, as they should be treated appropriately as per the condition.

Other causes

Other causes to rule out in fibromyalgia include:

- Infective causes: Lyme disease, hepatitis virus, HIV infections and, more recently, long COVID syndrome can mimic fibromyalgia.
- Metabolic abnormalities: diabetes and vitamin deficiencies need to be ruled out as they can present with a similar clinical picture of generalised weakness.

- Gastrointestinal disorders, such as coeliac disease and irritable bowel syndrome, can co-exist or mimic fibromyalgia.
- Malignancy: fatigue and widespread pain can mask the initial phase of malignancy. Other red flag symptoms, such as weight loss, night sweats or fever, should be addressed.
- Medications: statins, oncological medications, opioids and many other medications can cause widespread muscle pain and this needs to be considered. Approximately 2–10% of patients on statins can present with muscle pain. Opioid-induced allodynia is often difficult to diagnose, as these patients experience widespread pain; a trial of changing opioids or weaning off slowly might help in the diagnosis.

Underdiagnosis

It is claimed by some studies that fibromyalgia can be underdiagnosed to a significant extent. Physicians might lack the knowledge to diagnose correctly or might be hesitant to give a diagnostic label in many of these situations. Furthermore, traditional medical school teaching still focuses on the medical model in which a diagnosis and treatment approach is taken, rather than the biopsychosocial model for conditions such as fibromyalgia that lack a clear biomarker or cure. Some specialists might feel comfortable to give a different diagnostic label; for example, a rheumatologist might consider a sero-negative condition, whilst a psychiatrist might give a label of anxiety or depression.

Overdiagnosis and misdiagnosis

Sometimes, regional or localised pain can be wrongly labelled as fibromyalgia. Inflammatory diseases can be considered a fibromyalgia syndrome.

Key Points

- Muscular, rheumatological, neurological, endocrine and psychiatric problems should be ruled out before a diagnosis of fibromyalgia.
- Fibromyalgia is underdiagnosed to some extent.

References

1. Chakrabarty S, Zoorob R. Fibromyalgia. *Am Fam Physician* 2007; 76(2): 247-54.
2. Häuser W, Perrot S, Sommer C, *et al*. Diagnostic cofounders of chronic widespread pain: not always fibromyalgia. *Pain Rep* 2017; 2(3): e598.
3. Häuser W, Sarzi-Puttini P, Fitzcharles MA. Fibromyalgia syndrome: under-, over- and misdiagnosis. *Clin Exp Rheumatol* 2019; 37(1) Suppl 116: 90-7.

Fibromyalgia

Section 4

Education

Fibromyalgia

Chapter 17

Biopsychosocial model

Introduction

Long-term management of fibromyalgia syndrome is based on the biopsychosocial model. As in any other chronic illness, fibromyalgia affects individuals physically, mentally and socially. Therefore, it is prudent to adopt a holistic approach when planning for patient rehabilitation. The aim is to improve the patient's quality of life which can be achieved by using the biopsychosocial model.

The biopsychosocial model

Application of the biopsychosocial model allows a holistic consideration of the patient based on three domains:

- 'Bio': physiological impact of the disease, especially pain, fatigue and weakness.
- 'Psycho': patient's altered emotions, behaviours and beliefs due to chronic pain, as well as associated catastrophisation.
- 'Social': economic and financial, environmental, social (including family relationships), cultural and occupational impact of fibromyalgia.

The biopsychosocial model was first proposed by George Engel in 1977 for chronic conditions and its application has been extrapolated to patients with chronic pain conditions. Healthcare professionals are well trained to look after the 'biological' aspect of illness, whilst the 'psychological' aspect can usually be explored by chronic pain clinics. However, the healthcare system is ill prepared and ill equipped in terms of tackling the 'social' impact of fibromyalgia syndrome.

Evidence for the biopsychosocial pathway in fibromyalgia

A Norwegian research study on the biopsychosocial model using a patient-centred recovery-oriented programme showed that this pathway reduced uncertainties and brought a positive attitude. A follow-up after 1 year indicated a better recovery outcome and showed that patients experienced more good days on this pathway.

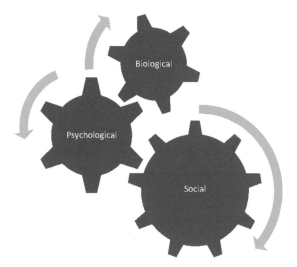

Figure 17.1. Biopsychosocial model in fibromyalgia syndrome.

Recent research from the USA categorising biopsychosocial factors concluded that health outcomes and life satisfaction differed significantly depending on the amount of biopsychosocial problems. This validated the need for biopsychosocial interventions for patients with fibromyalgia.

A biopsychosocial model in fibromyalgia syndrome is outlined in ▓ Figure 17.1.

Complex interactions in the biopsychosocial pathway

In the biopsychosocial pathway, functioning and disability have a complex interaction with the patient's biological conditions (pain, fatigue, etc.), psychological impact (anxiety, depression, brain fog) and social factors (contextual factors, social stigma). Fibromyalgia is a multilevel syndrome that encompasses all these factors.

Integration of the biopsychosocial model in fibromyalgia and pain management programmes

Biological, psychological and social factors all need to be considered together as a continuum. This approach will help in the planning of a comprehensive multidimensional, multimodal rehabilitation programme that is tailored specifically to a patient's individual needs.

Key Points

- A biopsychosocial model holds huge promise for taking an holistic approach in the management of fibromyalgia.
- All pain management approaches should encompass a biopsychosocial model as the basis for long-term management.

References

1.   Vasu T. The biopsychosocial model. In: Vasu T, Balasubramanian S, Kodivalasa M, Ingle PM, Eds. *Chronic pain management*. Shrewsbury, UK: tfm publishing Ltd; 2021: pp. 21-4.

2.   Engel GL. The need for a new medical model: a challenge for biomedicine. *Science* 1977; 196(4286): 129-36.

3.   Mengshoel AM, Skarbø Å, Hasselknippe E, *et al*. Enabling personal recovery from fibromyalgia – theoretical rationale, content, and meaning of a person-centred, recovery-oriented programme. *BMC Health Serv Res* 2021; 21(1): 339.

4.   Muller V, Chan F, Iwanaga K, *et al*. An empirically derived taxonomy of biopsychosocial factors of adjustment to fibromyalgia: results of a multivariate analysis. *Rehabil Couns Bull* 2020; 64(1): 3-16.

Chapter 18

Education

Introduction

Education is an important tool in any chronic condition management strategy; it is the first step in the comprehensive pain management plan in fibromyalgia. Unless the patient is educated regarding the diagnosis, aetiopathology and management strategies of fibromyalgia, it is impossible to create a rapport and engage with them in the treatment pathway. Many patients have lost their trust in the medical services and go through a 'revolving-door' phenomenon seeing many specialists with unsatisfactory outcomes as they are not educated about the disease. Without education, the health service cannot match the patient's expectations of the service with what it can deliver. Any fibromyalgia clinic should allocate adequate time to educate their patients, without which the service is doomed to fail these people.

Complexity of fibromyalgia

As we discussed in Chapters 5–10, the causation of fibromyalgia is very complex. It is not only difficult for patients, but it is also difficult in many circumstances to educate healthcare professionals. As mentioned in Chapter 12, many healthcare professionals consider fibromyalgia as 'the least prestigious disease' to have; this opinion might cause reluctance and apathy on the part of the clinician to educate patients.

Patients who are less informed about their disease can catastrophise more and might not engage in the management plan offered by the clinician. Education in pain neurophysiology can itself be considered a tool to tackle central sensitisation and help with the goal of 'keeping active'.

Health education

Education by qualified/trained clinicians leads to changes in the patient's health behaviour, leading to a change in their health status and improvement in their quality of life. Education helps to attain these goals by changing the patient's perception of the disease. In fibromyalgia, this can lead to the patient taking control of managing their condition themselves, rather than passively relying only on the healthcare system.

Education that fibromyalgia is a real disease

Many patients doubt themselves and question whether they are imagining the disease or if 'it is all in their brain'. It is important to inform them that the brain is the higher centre involved in the perception of pain and their pain is real. Education in neurophysiology can help them to understand their pain and also provide confidence that the clinician believes their symptoms. At the same time, it should be stressed that the best way to manage this complex neurophysiology is to use the biopsychosocial multimodal approach.

Biopsychosocial education

Traditional pain clinic education strategies look at a self-management pathway using the biopsychosocial model. Most clinics also incorporate cognitive behavioural, acceptance and commitment-based or mindfulness-based approaches. These approaches are used as individual educational strategies, or mixed with interventions or complementary therapies, or as a part of comprehensive rehabilitation-based pain management programmes.

Pain neuroscience education

Pain neuroscience education focuses on reconceptualising the origin of pain and helps patients to understand the aetiology, thereby leading to a change in their negative beliefs or cognitions regarding pain; this will lead to less pain catastrophisation. A randomised double-blinded trial showed that pain physiology education improved health status and endogenous pain inhibition in fibromyalgia. In this study, spatially accumulating thermal nociceptive stimuli were used as an evaluation tool to measure the efficacy of pain inhibitory mechanisms.

Supplementing educational advice with various media tools

Written material, such as leaflets, can engage patients in a better way to reinforce the principles of pain management in fibromyalgia. Technology advances, such as websites, apps, and various online platforms, should be used as these can promote educational tools in a more productive way.

Internet-based educational intervention

It is vital to harness the benefits of internet- and web-based approaches to deliver educational interventions in fibromyalgia. Due to the COVID-19 pandemic, many pain services that had never used web-based tools in the past also started using these approaches. Even after the pandemic stabilised, these services have continued to use these tools for patients with chronic pain with much benefit. An analysis of using a participatory approach in eHealth interventions in patients with fibromyalgia has shown it to be of benefit in enhancing the overall effectiveness and improving self-management strategies.

Evidence for education in fibromyalgia

A systematic analysis of a small group of studies on the effectiveness of education in fibromyalgia has shown that with education there was a significant reduction in the perception of the disease, catastrophisation, pain intensity and anxiety.

Biochemical evidence of education

A randomised trial showed that an 11-week education programme group experienced better outcomes than the control group. The study showed an improvement in the levels of cytokines (IL-4 plasma level, anti-inflammatory/inflammatory cytokine ratio) and cortisol (salivary cortisol levels) in the experimental group, proposing the idea that education can induce subjective (using Fibromyalgia Impact Questionnaire scores) and objective changes in the immune and neuroendocrine systems, and leading to improvement in health status in patients with fibromyalgia.

Cost-effectiveness of educational strategies

A randomised controlled trial of psychoeducation in patients with fibromyalgia showed that it produced significant long-term clinical effectiveness and cost-effectiveness. In this study, the education group showed improvement in global functional status and a better quality-adjusted life-year (QALY) score per person. At the same time, the mean incremental cost saved per person per year in the education group was €215.49 from the healthcare perspective and €197.32 from the societal perspective.

Comparison of education pathways

A double-blinded, randomised multicentre controlled clinical trial showed that for fibromyalgia that there was no difference between a written relaxation training education strategy and a written pain neuroscience training education strategy. Written material in the form of leaflets might consolidate the education from pain programmes, but their individual validity is questioned by this research.

Comparison of duration in pain neuroscience education

A study compared three different levels of education in pain neuroscience with that of a control group. The outcomes were measured in terms of conditioned pain modulation, temporal summation and pressure pain thresholds and followed up at 3 months. The study showed that the intensive pain neuroscience education produced a larger improvement in pain management.

Combination of exercise and education

A randomised trial compared exercise, education and their combination in a controlled manner in fibromyalgia. It concluded that the benefits of exercise were enhanced when combined with targeted self-management education. The study showed the benefits in improving functional status, key symptoms and self-efficacy; these benefits persisted during the 6-month duration of the study.

A systematic review in fibromyalgia has shown that patient education alone did not prove to be effective, but there was strong evidence that if education was combined with exercise and active coping strategies, it improved quality of life and functionality in the short, medium and long term. This study had a limitation of only including five randomised trials.

Difficulties in analysing educational tools

There is great heterogeneity in the educational approaches used by various healthcare services with regards to fibromyalgia. Each education session differed significantly from the other in duration, tools used, inclusive or exclusive criteria, and its content. This made it difficult to advise which educational approach was best; the goal should be to educate patients in neurophysiology, engage patients in self-management strategies and allow patients to take control of their pain.

Key Points

- Education is the first and vital step in a comprehensive management plan for fibromyalgia.
- Biopsychosocial education and pain neuroscience education are commonly used in clinical practice and have a good evidence base.
- Internet-based educational interventions have been used more recently in fibromyalgia with some success.
- The combination of exercise and education was found to be more effective in patients with fibromyalgia.

References

1. Album D, Westin S. Do diseases have a prestige hierarchy? A survey among physicians and medical students. *Soc Sci Med* 2008; 66(1): 182-8.

2. García-Ríos MC, Navarro-Ledesma S, Tapia-Haro RM, *et al.* Effectiveness of health education in patients with fibromyalgia: a systematic review. *Eur J Phys Rehabil Med* 2019; 55(2): 301-13.

3. van Oosterwijck J, Meeus M, Paul L, *et al.* Pain physiology education improves health status and endogenous pain inhibition in fibromyalgia. A double-blind randomized controlled trial. *Clin J Pain* 2013; 29(10): 873-82.

4. Camerini L, Camerini A, Schulz PJ. Do participation and personalization matter? A model-driven evaluation of an internet-based patient education intervention for fibromyalgia patients. *Patient Educ Couns* 2013; 92(2): 229-34.

5. Pereira Pernambuco A, de Souza Cota Carvalho L, Pereira Leite Schetino L, *et al.* Effects of a health education program on cytokines and cortisol levels in fibromyalgia patients: a randomized controlled trial. *Adv Rheumatol* 2018; 58(1): 21.

6. Luciano JV, Sabes-Figuera R, Cardeñosa E, *et al.* Cost-utility of a psychoeducational intervention in fibromyalgia patients compared with usual care: an economic evaluation alongside a 12-month randomized controlled trial. *Clin J Pain* 2013; 29(8): 702-11.

7. van Ittersum MW, van Wilgen CP, van der Schans CP, *et al.* Written pain neuroscience education in fibromyalgia: a multicenter randomized controlled trial. *Pain Pract* 2014; 14(8): 689-700.

8.   Rooks DS, Gautam S, Romeling M, *et al.* Group exercise, education, and combination self-management in women with fibromyalgia: a randomized trial. *Arch Intern Med* 2007; 167(20): 2192-200.

9.   Amer-Cuenca JJ, Pecos-Martín D, Martínez-Merinero P, *et al.* How much is needed? Comparison of the effectiveness of different pain education dosages in patients with fibromyalgia. *Pain Med* 2020; 21(4): 782-93.

10.   Elizagaray-Garcia I, Muriente-Gonzalez J, Gil-Martinez A. Education for patients with fibromyalgia. A systematic review of randomised clinical trials. *Rev Neurol* 2016; 62(2): 49-60.

Fibromyalgia

Chapter 19

Communication and building a rapport

Introduction

Communication is challenging for both patients and clinicians in fibromyalgia. A qualitative study showed that the most common recurring theme in fibromyalgia was dissatisfaction amongst both professionals and patients. Whilst clinicians expressed the frustration that they were of little help to their patients, patients expressed dissatisfaction with the delay in reaching a diagnosis and reported the need for greater moral support from their clinicians.

Difficulty in communicating

Patients with fibromyalgia experience 'brain fog', which includes problems with cognition, memory, thinking and concentration. This causes significant hindrance in expressing their feelings and in communicating with healthcare professionals, family and friends.

Furthermore, disbelief of their symptoms and a lack of understanding among clinicians and others surrounding them can lead to restricted communication. Having invisible symptoms makes it difficult for patients to express their problems and also for others surrounding them to understand their condition.

Healing skills of communication

Whilst talking and explaining on its own can be therapeutic, it can also reduce anxiety and provide comfort through education; it can also help indirectly by improving patient understanding and trust, leading to better compliance with treatment. One study showed increased adherence to treatment and better self-care skills; this will in turn improve patient health and well-being.

Key aspects of communication

It is vital to stress the basic principles of communication between a patient and a clinician, as published by the United States Institute of Medicine of the National Academies:

- Mutual respect between the patient and clinician.
- Harmonised goals: this should be the most important aspect in consultation with a patient with fibromyalgia; the clinician should believe the symptoms but clarify what the patient's goals are and what the clinic can achieve.
- Supportive environment: at least to make sure that patients express their concerns and are open to discussing their problems.
- Appropriate decision partners: skills and competence appropriate to the patient; the patient will then gain confidence in the services delivered.
- Right information: risks, benefits and alternative options to be detailed.
- Transparency: a clear acknowledgement of the limits of the service.
- Continuous learning: regular feedback between patients and clinicians.

Listening skills

Any clinician involved in managing patients with fibromyalgia should have good listening skills. Patients with fibromyalgia often complain that they are not heard and that clinicians do not listen to their problems. Given that these patients have undergone a complex journey going through various medical specialties focusing on the cure model, it is vital to listen and confirm back to them that the clinician understands their problem. It is important to summarise their history and repeat it back to the patient to confirm whether the understanding of the clinician is a fair reflection of the patient's emotional and physical pain.

Shared decision making

Shared decision making is considered a solution to improving the interaction between patients with fibromyalgia and healthcare providers. A randomised trial of shared decision making in patients with fibromyalgia showed the positive quality of the physician-patient interaction; this reduced frustration in these patients. Shared decision making can reduce the problems inherent in the paternalistic healthcare medical-based approach, and can increase the scope of informed patient choice. Apart from improving satisfaction and reducing conflicts, shared decision making can improve clinical outcomes in physiological, functional and subjective domains.

Cues and concerns during communication

A study of cues and concerns during communication with patients with fibromyalgia showed that a lack of empathetic responding was associated with more cues, whilst empathetic communication led to the expression of more concerns. During the consultations, patients might not express their concerns directly, and can express them indirectly as cues. Patient-centred communication can facilitate the expression and recognition of cues and concerns in patients with fibromyalgia.

Using metaphors in communication

The following chapter (Chapter 20) will specifically deal with the use of metaphors to improve communication in fibromyalgia. The author strongly recommends these strategies to improve the outcome of the clinics by a better patient understanding of the management pathways.

Key Points

- Communication can be challenging for both patients and clinicians.
- Brain fog can make it difficult for patients with fibromyalgia to express their feelings.
- Better communication can improve both compliance with treatment and self-care skills.
- Shared decision making between the patient and the clinician can improve outcomes in fibromyalgia.

References

1. Briones-Vozmediano E, Vives-Cases C, Ronda-Pérez E, Gil-González D. Patients' and professionals' views on managing fibromyalgia. *Pain Res Manag* 2013; 18(1): 19-24.

2. Street RL, Makoul G, Arora NK, Epstein RM. How does communication heal? Pathway linking clinician-patient communication to health outcomes. *Patient Educ Couns* 2009; 74(3): 295-301.

3. Paget L, Han P, Nedza S, *et al*. Patient-clinician communication: basic principles and expectations. Institute of Medicine of National Academies; June 2011. Available from: https://nam.edu/wp-content/uploads/2015/06/VSRT-Patient-Clinician.pdf.

4. Bieber C, Müller KG, Blumenstiel K, *et al*. A shared decision-making communication training program for physicians treating fibromyalgia patients: effects of a randomized controlled trial. *J Psychosom Res* 2008; 64(1): 13-20.

5. Eide H, Sibbern T, Egeland T, *et al*. Fibromyalgia patients' communication of cues and concerns: interaction analysis of pain clinic consultations. *Clin J Pain* 2011; 27(7): 602-10.

Chapter 20

Using metaphors to communicate

Introduction

A metaphor is a figure of speech in which a word or phrase denoting one kind of object or idea is used in place of another to suggest a likeness or analogy between them. It comes from the Greek word 'metaphora' meaning 'to transfer'. Fibromyalgia is a complex pain condition with an unclear aetiology and undefined treatment pathways; the patient is compromised enormously due to a lack of understanding of the condition and abnormal fear or catastrophisation. This leads to a vicious cycle of a worsening pain state. There is clear evidence that a better understanding of pain neurophysiology changes pain cognition and physical performance; using metaphors can be very effective in achieving these goals in fibromyalgia.

Mechanism of effectiveness

Pain neurophysiology is complex, especially in chronic pain conditions. Using metaphors can simplify the explanation and can transfer the meaning effectively in fibromyalgia. It further clarifies the message to the patients that the clinician believes that their pain is real and has an understanding of the physiology behind their painful condition.

Inappropriate use of metaphors

In clinical practice, many clinicians already use metaphors inappropriately. Metaphors of 'crumbling spine' or 'fighting against fibromyalgia' can communicate a negative image of the patient's understanding of pain; this can lead to further catastrophising and persistent pain illness behaviour. Educating the clinician in the use of appropriate words and metaphors in the fibromyalgia clinic can reduce these disasters and can improve outcomes.

Differentiating acute and chronic pain

Without metaphors it is a struggle to differentiate the mechanisms of acute versus chronic pain in a patient with fibromyalgia. Using the metaphor of an alarm system that has gone haywire can easily explain why some pain is chronic. This differentiates the pain neuromatrix system from the traditional pain pathways, as this might be difficult even for some healthcare professionals to understand.

Metaphors allow patients to express themselves better

A qualitative study of women with fibromyalgia showed that metaphors helped to explore the lived experience by creative data expression methods. Metaphorical representation allowed these patients to express a holistic view of their fibromyalgia experience. Using the metaphor of journeys between health and illness was a common narrative described in this study.

Evidence for metaphors

Randomised controlled trials have shown that a booklet of metaphors and stories conveying pain biology concepts can assist in reconceptualising pain and reducing catastrophisation. Studies have found that these changes were maintained for at least 3 months.

Acceptance and commitment therapy

Newer psychological approaches such as acceptance and commitment therapy (ACT) uses an acceptance and mindfulness approach, combined with a commitment and behavioural change process. Metaphors are vital to this approach, lead to better acceptance and aid the patient's commitment to changes.

Problems with metaphors

A clinician needs the skill and expertise to use the right metaphor at the right time in the right context. It has to be targeted to the right patient in the right way. If the meaning of the metaphor and the context is not understood by the patient, this can lead to further confusion. Prior assessment of patient understanding and appropriateness is vital before using the metaphor tool. A metaphor cannot stand on its own and the clinician has to verify that the meaning has been expressed clearly; this could be confirmed and checked by making sure that the patient has understood the metaphor, rather than its meaning being lost in translation. Once a clinician has gained more experience in applying metaphors, their use can become routine practice in their armamentarium for managing fibromyalgia.

Key Points

- Metaphors are used in pain neuroscience education in fibromyalgia.
- Metaphors can reduce pain catastrophising and lead to a better understanding of the condition.
- Metaphors are commonly used to differentiate and explain the pain neuromatrix physiology.
- Patients with fibromyalgia can use metaphors to express their emotions in a better way.
- It is vital that the clinician uses metaphors appropriately and that the meaning is not lost in translation in the clinical context.

References

1.   Definition of metaphor. Available from: http://www.merriam-webster.com/dictionary/metaphor.

2.   Moseley GL, Nicholas MK, Hodges PW. A randomized controlled trial of intensive neurophysiology education in chronic low back pain. *Clin J Pain* 2004; 20(5): 324-30.

3.   Brown N, Vougioukalou SA. Exploring the lived experience of fibromyalgia using creative data collection methods. *Cogent Soc Sci* 2018; 4(1): 1447759.

4.   Gallagher L, McAuley J, Moseley GL. A randomized-controlled trial of using a book of metaphors to reconceptualize pain and decrease catastrophizing in people with chronic pain. *Clin J Pain* 2013; 29(1): 20-5.

Chapter 21

Patients taking control

Introduction

It is vital in any chronic condition such as fibromyalgia that the patient takes control of its management into their own hands, rather than leaving it passively in the hands of the healthcare professional. Scientific evidence has clearly shown that active self-management produces better outcomes than passive dependency.

The patient taking control of their pain versus the pain taking control of the patient

Most patients presenting to chronic pain clinics will tell the clinician that the fibromyalgia takes control of their lives! Using an acceptance and commitment approach, it is wise to suggest that the patient should take control of the pain and other symptoms, rather than letting the disease take control of their lives.

How to introduce the concept?

Letting the pain take control of their lives has happened up to now, and it is appropriate to use the correct metaphors and question whether this approach has led to any success. Most, or all, patients will clearly say that it has not. Challenges need to be introduced to determine whether the patient wants to look at this with a slightly different approach, although this does not mean that there is a magic wand to erase the pain.

Being an active partner

Patients with chronic conditions should be active partners in managing their condition. Leaving the control of their condition in the hands of the clinician leads to poorer outcomes. The clinician should guide and provide the correct skills and confidence to patients to let them be active managers of their own health.

Self-management

Self-management refers to the ability of the patient to monitor their fibromyalgia and affect the behavioural, cognitive and emotional responses, in order to have a satisfactory quality of life. It helps to develop, apply and maintain the appropriate skills in patients with fibromyalgia in their everyday life. Self-management should be focused in a multidimensional way.

Components of self-management

It is unfortunate that all fibromyalgia programmes vary in how they promote self-management; there is no standardisation of strategies used and so it is difficult to find the appropriate evidence. Lorig and Holman have defined self-management as consisting of three tasks: medical management, role management and emotional management. They further classify six important skills: problem solving, decision making, resource utilisation, forming a partnership with the provider, action planning and self-tailoring.

Evidence for self-management strategies

A meta-analysis of 39 studies showed that self-management strategies improved physical function and pain over short- and long-term durations in patients with fibromyalgia. Studies from the Stanford Patient Education Research Center, looking at chronic conditions, showed improved behaviours in a follow-up of 1–4 years. A randomised controlled trial of an outpatient multidisciplinary programme for fibromyalgia proved that self-management strategies improved the quality of life and that the functional consequences were persistent even 6 months after the completion of the programme. Another study showed that the benefits of exercise were enhanced when combined with targeted self-management education.

How can clinicians help with self-management strategies?

The focus of chronic pain management in fibromyalgia should be self-management strategies; any treatment programme without this foundation will fail. It has been shown that self-management strategies do not develop as one uniform pattern; these behaviours can develop in various patterns including consistent, episodic, on demand and transitional. The clinician should support self-management strategies tailored to each patient's behaviour development pattern.

Barriers to self-management

Illness catastrophising is the main barrier to self-management and recovery in fibromyalgia; the appropriate explanation and education are the keys to overcoming this hurdle. However, studies have shown that ethnic grouping, financially vulnerable conditions, comorbidities, low self-efficacy and demanding social obligations can all be significant barriers to self-management strategies.

Key Points

- It is important for patients with fibromyalgia to take control of their condition in their hands rather than expecting passive treatments alone.
- Clinicians should guide and provide the correct skills and confidence to patients so that they can take on the role of active managers of their own health.
- Self-management develops, applies and maintains appropriate skills in the everyday lives of these patients.
- Illness catastrophising can hinder these strategies; appropriate explanation and education are the keys to recovery.

References

1. Barlow J, Wright C, Sheasby J, et al. Self-management approaches for people with chronic conditions: a review. Patient Educ Couns 2002; 48(2): 177-87.

2. Lorig KR, Holman HR. Self-management education: history, definition, outcomes, and mechanisms. Ann Behav Med 2003; 26(1): 1-7.

3. Geraghty AWA, Maund E, Newell D, et al. Self-management for chronic widespread pain including fibromyalgia: a systematic review and meta-analysis. PLoS ONE 2021; 16(7): e0254642.

4. Cedraschi C, Desmeules J, Rapiti E, et al. Fibromyalgia: a randomised, controlled trial of a treatment programme based on self management. Ann Rheum Dis 2004; 63(3): 290-6.

5. Rooks DS, Gautam S, Romeling M, et al. Group exercise, education, and combination self-management in women with fibromyalgia: a randomized trial. Arch Intern Med 2007; 167(20): 2192-200.

6. Audulv Å. The over time development of chronic illness self-management patterns: a longitudinal qualitative study. BMC Public Health 2013; 13: 452.

Chapter 22

Networking in fibromyalgia

Introduction

Patient support groups and networking play important roles for patients with fibromyalgia towards understanding their condition and accepting and committing to the management strategies, with the aim of looking for available treatments or services in their locality. Support and networking give them the confidence to engage in the self-management pathway to ensure the long-term management of their condition. It can help in the acceptance of the diagnosis and creates a greater understanding of the illness.

Patient support groups

In developed countries, such as the UK and the USA, there are patient support groups for fibromyalgia in most localities. These groups help the patients, as well as lobby for resources to help them. Most of these groups are run by the patients themselves, but some are appropriately guided by clinicians including their pain management teams. Social support groups and networking can help these patients to take control of the condition over a shorter time period and help to improve their quality of life. These groups can provide information, guidance, advice and direction on the right treatment option, but also provide emotional support from peers. The acceptability and compliance of treatment are higher, as the advice comes from peers who have had a similar experience.

Role of networking in illness acceptance

Qualitative research in long-term patients with fibromyalgia has shown that peer support groups can help in illness acceptance, as it can take a long time before the patient accepts their diagnosis. Peer support is seen as an impetus to an ongoing process of reconstruction of identity and helps patients to cope with fibromyalgia.

Fibromyalgia groups in the UK

Fibromyalgia Action UK (FMA UK) is a UK charity with the aim to raise awareness of fibromyalgia; it has various regional groups and supports with information regarding the condition.

UK Fibromyalgia claims to be an independent voice of UK patients with fibromyalgia. It provides information to create awareness and support the condition; it also publishes *Fibromyalgia Magazine.*

Fibromyalgia Friends Together is a support group for people with fibromyalgia and their carers, family and friends, and is based in Leicestershire. At the time of publication of this book, their website quoted that they met every third Thursday of the month, listen to people and help them come to terms with their illness.

Fibromyalgia Research UK is a patient support group that also runs a Facebook group with the aim of providing more information on the disease.

There are various online support groups both in the UK as well as all over the world; as these sites are not controlled, the quality and content cannot be guaranteed.

Many tertiary hospitals also run a local patient-run support group, many of which are part of the follow-up after their pain management programmes.

Fibromyalgia groups in the USA

The National Fibromyalgia Association (NFA) is a non-profit organisation with the aim of improving the quality of life for people with fibromyalgia. It assists local support groups and provides patient information and education. It publishes a magazine called *Fibromyalgia AWARE*. It has proclaimed the 12th of May as 'Fibromyalgia Awareness Day' and campaigns for the condition. It also supports research into the condition.

The National Fibromyalgia & Chronic Pain Association (NFMCPA) is an American association that supports patients with fibromyalgia. Since 1998, it has embraced the 12th of May as Fibromyalgia Awareness Day to create awareness of the condition. It has a Facebook page with more than 173,000 followers.

Living with Fibromyalgia (livingwithfibro.org) is a group that supports the community for fibromyalgia.

Support Fibromyalgia is another patient-centred non-profit organisation to educate and inspire the fibromyalgia community.

Most states have a local fibromyalgia support group that can be found and accessed via the internet.

Fibromyalgia groups in Canada

Fibromyalgia Association Canada aims to bring together people with fibromyalgia across Canada; it also wants to strengthen their presence and influence the government decision-makers regarding their healthcare.

There are various support groups, as in any other country, for fibromyalgia in each locality and province. Details are available from the above association's website.

Fibromyalgia groups in Australia

Fibromyalgia Australia aims to fast track the improvement of medical healthcare for Australians living with fibromyalgia.

Musculoskeletal Australia runs peer support groups for various conditions affecting the musculoskeletal system, including fibromyalgia.

Fibromyalgia groups in developing countries

It is possible to find various patient support groups for fibromyalgia through Facebook, Twitter and other social media, although these are less formally organised in developing countries.

Need and importance of networking among patients

Fibromyalgia is a challenging, complex condition; patients need a high level of commitment to manage this condition. Patient empowerment can not be fully achieved by the healthcare system alone; peer social support, if directed appropriately, can play a major role in managing this condition. It also helps to engage the patient in the biopsychosocial model of recovery. See Chapter 66 for more details on patient support groups and forums.

A qualitative study has shown that peer social support in women with fibromyalgia exerts positive effects on their physical, mental and social well-being and empowers them to manage their disease. This study showed that these networking opportunities increased the personal feelings of satisfaction in patients by creating greater well-being.

Key Points

- Patient support groups and networking play important roles in fibromyalgia with the aim to promote self-management strategies.
- Peer support groups, under the right guidance, can help in illness acceptance.
- Each country and locality has a fibromyalgia support group; clinicians should guide patients in the right direction to engage in these groups.
- Networking can improve physical, mental and social well-being among individuals with fibromyalgia.

References

1.   Sallinen M, Kukkurainen ML, Peltokallio L. Finally heard, believed and accepted – peer support in the narratives of women with fibromyalgia. *Patient Educ Couns* 2011; 85(2): e126-30.

2.   Fibromyalgia Action UK. Available from: https://www.fmauk.org/.

3.   UK Fibromyalgia: the Independent Voice of UK Fibromyalgia. Available from: https://ukfibromyalgia.com/.

4.   Fibromyalgia Friends Together. Available from: https://www.fibro.org.uk/support/.

5.   National Fibromyalgia Association. Available from: https://www.fmaware.org/.

6.   Support Fibromyalgia. Available from: https://supportfibromyalgia.org/.

7.   Fibromyalgia Association Canada. Available from: https://fibrocanada.ca/en/.

8.   Fibromyalgia Association Canada. Fibromyalgia support groups across Canada. Available from: https://fibrocanada.ca/en/resources/fm-support-groups-across-canada/.

9.   Fibromyalgia Australia. Available from: https://fibromyalgiaaustralia.org.au/.

10.   Musculoskeletal Australia. Peer support groups. Available from: https://msk.org.au/peer-support-groups/.

11.   Reig-Garcia G, Bosch-Farré C, Suñer-Soler R, *et al.* The impact of a peer social support network form the perspective of women with fibromyalgia: a qualitative study. *Int J Environ Res Public Health* 2021; 18(23): 12801.

Fibromyalgia

Chapter 23

Social media and fibromyalgia

Introduction

Social media can influence a health condition in both positive and negative ways; the healthcare professional can direct the patient with fibromyalgia to the right social media pathway, so he/she receives the correct messages to engage in the recovery pathway.

Social media use in fibromyalgia

Studies have shown that the use of social media is more frequent in patients with fibromyalgia. However, there was no relationship between the rates of social media use and the severity or prevalence of the disease.

Fibromyalgia Action UK undertook a survey in 2018 to understand the preferences of people with fibromyalgia with regards to social media platforms. The survey highlighted the need to use more visually engaging content to inform and educate individuals regarding the condition. The respondent demographics highlighted the limited interaction of younger people under the age of 35 with social media. The association started a new campaign titled #BecomeFibroAware, which uses visual content and has an increasing focus on younger people with fibromyalgia.

Information seeking during the illness

An online survey of patients with fibromyalgia showed that the respondents used the internet most frequently. Among the online resources, the most frequently used were the organisation websites, health portals and health-related social networking sites. The topics that were sought varied during the course of the illness.

Youtube

A study on fibromyalgia checked 200 videos against the guidelines from the American College of Rheumatology; the majority of the videos were presented by healthcare professionals (61.5%). This research concluded that most of the published videos did not follow the information recommended by the American College of Rheumatology. The authors concluded that the videos should be interpreted with caution and were not the most appropriate resource for health education on fibromyalgia.

Instagram

The fibromyalgia community is developing on Instagram; studies have shown that this platform can support the community of people with this condition. Instagram facilitates intimate and supportive interactions on the illness and creates personalised day-to-day narratives that are accessible to all.

Twitter

Twitter is a widely used social networking and microblogging service that generates huge numbers of communities of patients with fibromyalgia and their carers. It helps to vent frustration among patients; it can also help them to identify and validate their symptoms.

Research has been carried out using a content analysis of the information on Twitter to gain valuable insight into variations in fibromyalgia first-person experiences. The association between weather conditions and fibromyalgia symptoms was examined in a specific study using Twitter content, as these tweets contain huge amounts of additional data including date, time and location.

Facebook

An electronic survey involving a validated social support scale was conducted on a Facebook fibromyalgia community with more than 8000 members. The online environment was often indicated by these members as the place to vent feelings openly. Social discrimination was recorded on Facebook — from family, friends and even healthcare professionals. The study concluded that the new forms of online education and social support for fibromyalgia from online groups should be considered in patient care programmes.

Key Points

- The use of social media is high in patients with fibromyalgia.
- The information that patients seek varies during the course of the illness.
- YouTube, Instagram, Twitter and Facebook help to form a community for these patients.
- Social media also helps to vent feelings and provides identity and validation to patients with fibromyalgia.

References

1. Külekçioğlu S, Çetin A. Social media use in patients with fibromyalgia and its effect on symptom severity and sleep quality. *Adv Rheumatol* 2021; 61(1): 51.

2. Stones S, Henderson R, Quinn D. PARE0005 Refreshing the social media strategy of fibromyalgia action UK: results of a national patient organisation survey. *Ann Rheum Dis* 2019; 78: 2179.

3. Chen AT. Information seeking over the course of illness: the experience of people with fibromyalgia. *Musculoskelet Care* 2012; 10(4): 212-20.

4. Macedo CC, Figueiredo PHS, Gonçalves NRB, *et al*. Fibromyalgia in social media: content and quality of the information analysis of videos on the YouTube platform. *Inform Health Soc Care* 2021: 1-12.

5. Berard AA, Smith AP. Post your journey: Instagram as a support community for people with fibromyalgia. *Qual Health Res* 2019; 29(2): 237-47.

6. Delir Haghighi PD, Kang YB, Buchbinder R, *et al*. Investigating subjective experience and the influence of weather among individuals with fibromyalgia: a content analysis of Twitter. *JMIR Public Health Surveill* 2017; 3(1): e4.

7. Moretti FA, Silva SS, Novoa CG. Characteristics and perception of social support by patients with fibromyalgia in Facebook. *Br J Pain* 2018; 1(1): 4-8.

Section**5**

Physical therapies

Fibromyalgia

Chapter 24

Physical therapy

Introduction

Physiotherapists form a vital part of any pain management team. The Core Standards for Pain Management Services in the UK recommend that any pain service should include a Health & Care Professions Council (HCPC) registered physiotherapist. The standards also suggest that they should be additionally trained in cognitive behavioural therapy (CBT) principles of pain management. Most experienced physiotherapists also have expertise in acceptance and commitment therapy (ACT), mindfulness-based approaches and motivational interviewing techniques.

Physiotherapists in fibromyalgia

Physiotherapists play a valuable role in various aspects of fibromyalgia management:

- Education: allays anxiety and reduces pain catastrophising; this helps patients to take control of their own pain and engage in self-management pathways. Changing behavioural patterns can be the key to engaging with recovery pathways.
- Gradual exercises: it is essential that movements are performed gradually to prevent flare-up and fatigue; physiotherapists are well

positioned to assess and guide appropriately in this regard. It should be clearly explained that 'hurt does not mean harm', but at the same time the level of activity that is appropriate should be assessed, to prevent worsening of fatigue or flare-up.

- Complementary therapies: most trained physiotherapists also provide acupuncture, a transcutaneous electrical nerve stimulation (TENS) machine and other complementary therapies to help in recovery. Pain management programmes can also include yoga, tai chi and mindfulness-based breathing exercises that are delivered by physiotherapists.

- Desensitisation strategies, distraction and relaxation strategies are commonly used by physiotherapists as needed.

Evidence for physical therapy

The European League Against Rheumatism (EULAR) has recently revised its recommendations for the management of fibromyalgia (2017), and systematically reviewed 275 scientific papers and 107 reviews with a multidisciplinary group from 12 countries. This review clearly directed that the only 'strong for' therapy-based recommendation was exercise. It recommended a graduated approach for exercise. However, these guidelines clarified that there was no evidence to distinguish between aerobic and strengthening exercises.

Other national guidelines

In April 2017, the German Pain Society coordinated and published guidelines with the interaction of 13 scientific societies and two patient self-help organisations. They strongly recommended low-to-moderate intensity endurance and strength training for fibromyalgia. They concluded that chiropractic, laser therapy, magnetic field therapy, massage and transcranial magnetic stimulation were not recommended.

Other evidence for physiotherapy

A randomised trial of patients with fibromyalgia with a 6-month follow-up showed that physiotherapy was similar in benefit to taking amitriptyline, with regards to disability reduction and improving outcome.

Aerobic exercise in fibromyalgia

Aerobic exercises are rhythmic, moderate-intensity activities such as walking, cycling and swimming that increase the respiratory rate and heart rate; they improve the cardiovascular status and help to control body weight.

A Cochrane review on aerobic exercise training in fibromyalgia studied 13 randomised controlled trials (RCTs); moderate-quality evidence indicated that aerobic exercise probably improved health-related quality of life. Low-quality evidence suggested that aerobic exercise may slightly decrease pain intensity and may slightly improve physical function. Aerobic exercise did not improve fatigue. However, the long-term effects of aerobic exercise showed little or no difference.

Resistance and strengthening exercises

Resistance and strengthening exercises improved strength, for example, lifting weights. These need to be planned appropriately, as they can worsen pain and fatigue in patients with fibromyalgia.

If done gradually, these exercises can improve the function and mood of patients.

A randomised trial of kinesiotherapy and stretching exercises showed that both improved flexibility levels and general well-being of women with fibromyalgia.

Relaxation techniques

Physiotherapists are experts in teaching the right relaxation strategies down an appropriate pathway for patients with fibromyalgia. Stress has a direct link with symptoms in fibromyalgia; regular relaxation strategies will help in the better management of the condition.

Positive experience

Qualitative research has shown that an appropriate physiotherapy programme in a group setting can lead to positive experiences of the body, as well as sharing experiences of living with fibromyalgia and creating new patterns of behaviour; the authors described this as an embodied learning process.

Key Points

- Physiotherapists play a vital role in the recovery of patients with fibromyalgia; they educate and reduce pain catastrophising in these patients.
- EULAR guidelines have only one 'strong for' recommendation: gradual exercise.
- Physiotherapy can improve the well-being and mood in patients with fibromyalgia.

References

1. Faculty of Pain Medicine of the Royal College of Anaesthetists. Core standards for pain management services in the UK. Available from: https://fpm.ac.uk/standards-publications-workforce/core-standards.

2. Macfarlane GJ, Kronisch C, Dean LE, *et al.* EULAR revised recommendations for the management of fibromyalgia. *Ann Rheum Dis* 2017; 76(2): 318-28.

3. Winkelmann A, Bork H, Brückle W, *et al.* Physiotherapy, occupational therapy and physical therapy in fibromyalgia syndrome: updated guidelines 2017 and overview of systematic review articles. *Schmerz* 2017; 31(3): 255-65.

4. Joshi MN, Joshi R, Jain AP. Effect of amitriptyline vs. physiotherapy in management of fibromyalgia syndrome: what predicts a clinical benefit? *J Postgrad Med* 2009; 55(3): 185-9.

5. Bidonde J, Busch AJ, Schachter CL, *et al.* Aerobic exercise training for adults with fibromyalgia. *Cochrane Database Syst Rev* 2017; 6(6): CD012700.

6. Valencia M, Alonso B, Alvarez MJ, *et al.* Effects of 2 physiotherapy programs on pain perception, muscular flexibility, and illness impact in women with fibromyalgia: a pilot study. *J Manipulative Physiol Ther* 2009; 32(1): 84-92.

7. National Health Service. Self-help – fibromyalgia. Available from: https://www.nhs.uk/conditions/fibromyalgia/self-help/.

8. Mannerkorpi K, Gard G. Physiotherapy group treatment for patients with fibromyalgia – an embodied learning process. *Disabil Rehabil* 2003; 25(24): 1372-80.

Fibromyalgia

Chapter 25

Pacing strategies

Introduction

Pacing involves balancing periods of activity with periods of rest, and not overdoing activities or pushing oneself beyond the limits. If not paced, patients with fibromyalgia can experience post-exertional fatigue and worsening pain.

Evidence for pacing

A systematic review of 41 studies has shown that both avoidance of activity and overactivity are associated with poorer patient outcomes. This study stressed the need for pacing and concluded that pacing is linked to better physiological functioning.

A Dutch survey of 409 patients with fibromyalgia concluded that active avoidance including guarding and asking for assistance was associated with disabilities, whilst pacing was not. The study proved the fear-avoidance model and suggested that specific active avoidance behaviours could be detrimental in fibromyalgia.

Techniques of pacing

Patients are better starting with low levels of activity and gradually increasing their activity, whilst making sure it is also balanced with time for recovery. These periods of rest give time to allow the patient to recuperate, rather than becoming overwhelmed with symptoms. Gradual increases should be well planned and can be targeted in very small increments over days or weeks.

Gentle exercises and breathing exercises can be started with a mindfulness approach, before proceeding to aerobic or strengthening exercises.

For patients with fibromyalgia, there are no specific exercises to avoid but, at the same time, it is vital that patients pace any mode of exercise.

Steps in pacing

Pacing involves various steps including:

- Setting the baseline: this needs a proper evaluation, as this is the basis on which pacing can start. A good physiotherapist can guide this, but always with full active agreement from the patient.
- Smaller regular chunks of activity: it is better to plan to break the activities into smaller chunks, but this should be done regularly.
- Gradual increments: the baseline should be practised for at least a week and then, if any increment is to be applied, it can be only 10% or less, and this should be planned well in advance. Each incremental increase should have a gap of 1 week in between.
- Setting goals: these goals should involve the personal interest of the patient. Goals that are achievable should be the focus, so that the patient can gain more confidence in the process.

Using metaphors for energy pacing

Rather than activity, the health professional can talk of energy pacing so that the patient understands the emotional component of this pacing strategy rather than the physical part alone. Using the 'tortoise and hare' fable can help to reiterate that 'slow and steady will win the race' at the end, despite some possible hiccups along the way. Explaining the vicious cycle of pain, distress, muscle fatigue and the need to break this cycle is often explained in many fibromyalgia programmes. Using the elastic band analogy to explain that muscles that have not been used and deconditioned for a long time, can take effort and time to get back to normal can help some patients. Always the message of 'hurt does not mean harm' should be given after making sure that all other causes are ruled out.

Prioritising tasks

Working smarter by prioritising tasks that are important and when to do them during the day is a vital part to success in the pacing strategy. A patient with fibromyalgia will be very keen to do all the activities that are wished for, but a clear discussion is needed with the physiotherapist at the start regarding what priorities are important. Of course, other activities and needs can be gradually and slowly built into the pacing plan with active involvement of the patient.

Step-down does not mean failure

The patient with fibromyalgia might need to step down from their activity level if there is a significant post-exertional flare-up of pain or fatigue. This is not a failure, but the message that the body is giving to the patient to reduce the activity further. Confidence must be given, and the baseline or activity level should be reduced, but a gradual step-up should be planned; slow, gradual increments are key to a pacing plan.

Methods of pacing

Operant learned pacing uses quotas related to time or goals that the patient sets; this is goal- or time-contingent, rather than focusing on pain, and are gradually increased using 'activity-rest' cycling. Energy conservation pacing uses the energy expenditure of the patient to pace themselves; the aim is to avoid pain and fatigue. A randomised trial has shown that operant learning might be more beneficial than energy conservation and could be an effective stand-alone activity for pacing treatment for patients with fibromyalgia.

Key Points

- Pacing balances periods of activity with periods of rest, so that the patient with fibromyalgia is not overexerted and does not experience fatigue or pain.
- Setting baseline and gradual increments are the key to pacing.
- It might be tempting for patients with fibromyalgia to do more exercise, but prioritising and setting goals are vital.
- With regards to strategies for pacing, operant learning might be more beneficial than energy conservation.

References

1.   Andrews NE, Strong J, Meredith PJ. Activity pacing, avoidance, endurance, and associations with patient functioning in chronic pain: a systematic review and meta-analysis. *Arch Phys Med Rehabil* 2012; 93(11): 2109-2121.e7.

2.   Karsdorp PA, Vlaeyen JWS. Active avoidance but not activity pacing is associated with disability in fibromyalgia. *Pain* 2009; 147(1-3): 29-35.

3.   National Health Service. Self-help – fibromyalgia. Available from: https://www.nhs.uk/conditions/fibromyalgia/self-help/.

4.   Racine M, Jensen MP, Harth M, *et al.* Operant learning versus energy conservation activity pacing treatments in a sample of patients with fibromyalgia syndrome: a pilot randomized controlled trial. *J Pain* 2019; 20(4): 420-39.

Chapter 26

Role of the occupational therapist

Introduction

As chronic pain is always managed with a biopsychosocial perspective, the role of the occupational therapist is important in multidisciplinary management. Assessment and interventional strategies by an occupational therapist can be done in a hospital, community or work setting. Many patients with fibromyalgia even struggle with their day-to-day activities such as washing and dressing; the occupational therapist aids these patients in their clinical recovery.

Pathway in the occupational therapy clinic

A detailed consultation made up of an interview and assessment helps the clinician to create an occupational profile; specific standardised occupational performance measures are used as practised in the setting. This approach helps to identify problems with the patient and the clinician can then guide them to set collaborative goals. The occupational therapist focuses on creating key performance areas that are meaningful to the patient.

Assessment by the occupational therapist

Assessment is done globally in various domains including:

- Day-to-day chores and activities.
- Essential activities such as washing and dressing.
- Cognitive assessment.
- Workplace: seating, wheelchair and mobility issues.
- Workplace ergonomics.
- Functional assessment.
- Need for aids and adaptations.
- Risk assessment.
- Social interactions and adaptations.

Tasks from the occupational therapist

The therapy session lasts over a few weeks and the therapist guides the patient to carry out various activities within the comprehensive recovery plan made collaboratively. These could include:

- Instruction for pacing in the workplace or setting a timetable for gradual cohesion with the role.
- Instruction and planning pacing with regards to household chores.
- Pacing with exercise, which will start with baseline identification, prioritisation and going slow.
- Advice on posture and body mechanics during the tasks.
- Some occupational therapists are also trained in psychological strategies including mindfulness.
- Occupational therapists can direct patients to online tools and community groups to engage patients in self-management strategies.
- Occupational therapists can be an active part of the group pain management programmes.

Evidence for occupational therapy

Poole and Siegel carried out a systematic review. They found that strong evidence was reported for some therapies offered by occupational therapists, including cognitive behavioural interventions, relaxation and stress management, emotional disclosure, physical activity and multidisciplinary interventions. However, these treatments are a spectrum offered by different specialists from the multidisciplinary team with an overlap of therapies between these specialists.

Self-management education with occupational therapists

A scientific study on occupational therapy-led motivational interviewing and mindfulness-based cognitive therapy in patients with fibromyalgia was shown to be highly effective in achieving health behaviour change, shifting patients' awareness and reducing relapse over the long term. Motivational interviewing is a patient-centred, directive counselling approach used to change health behaviours in patients with fibromyalgia.

Similar self-management support in a group setting for 6 weeks was highly beneficial, based on qualitative studies. However, as mentioned earlier, these therapies overlap with various other specialties and group pain management programmes are usually offered with multiple specialists in a multidisciplinary setting.

Occupational therapists and recovery

Fibromyalgia can cause challenges for the patient when they try to return to work; occupational therapists can help with this challenge and guide the patient on their pathway to recovery. The aim of consultations and interventions by occupational therapists should be to gain as much independence as possible and improve the quality of life for the patient with fibromyalgia.

Key Points

- Many patients with fibromyalgia can have restrictions in simple activities such as washing, dressing and cooking; occupational therapy helps in the day-to-day task performance of these individuals.
- Workplace assessment, changes and adaptations can be carried out by the occupational therapist to aid the patient in planning their recovery and engagement in their job.
- In fibromyalgia, the evidence for occupational therapy is available for many interventions, but these overlap with other specialties in the multidisciplinary group.

References

1. Siegel P, Jones BL, Poole JL. Occupational therapy interventions for adults with fibromyalgia. *Am J Occup Ther* 2018; 72(5): 7205395010p1-4.

2. Poole JL, Siegel P. Effectiveness of occupational therapy interventions for adults with fibromyalgia: a systematic review. *Am J Occup Ther* 2017; 71(1): 7101180040p1-10.

3. Prior Y, Walker N. Rheumatology occupational therapy-led fibromyalgia self-management education using motivational interviewing and mindfulness based cognitive therapy: a new approach. *Br J Occup Ther* 2016; 30(1): 8-13.

4. Corless L, Ching A, Mayana K, *et al*. 052 Occupational therapy-led fibromyalgia self-management education group programme: patients' perspectives. *Rheumatology* 2019; 58(Supplement_3): kez106.051.

Chapter 27

Functional rehabilitation programmes

Introduction

Various programmes for fibromyalgia exist with regards to planning for recovery and rehabilitation; details of pain management programmes commonly practised in the UK are given in Chapter 60. Graded exercise programmes are described in Chapter 28. This chapter details physiotherapy and occupational therapy-based functional rehabilitation programmes.

Functional impairment in fibromyalgia

Fibromyalgia significantly affects functional performance, both in day-to-day tasks and complex tasks. One study assessed functional impairment in female patients with fibromyalgia and compared them with a control group; it concluded that patients with fibromyalgia had significant impairment in both gait and balance. Walking speed was diminished due to both reduction in stride length and cycle frequency. Differences were significant for balance due to body sway in the medial-lateral and anterior-posterior axes. This suggested that fibromyalgia rehabilitation for physical impairment of postural control and gait is as important as the psychological response to pain.

Functional rehabilitation

Functional rehabilitation aims to help patients with fibromyalgia to return to their maximum possible levels of independence in activities that are important to them. The goals of any intervention vary depending on the priorities and abilities of the patient. These might vary diversely from some patients aiming to do their day-to-day activities such as washing and dressing to some planning active exercise and engaging in their occupation.

Pre-requisites for functional rehabilitation

The target in functional rehabilitation is improved function, and not reduction in pain; however, pain usually improves once function is recovered. The patient should be evaluated carefully and both patient and clinician should be convinced that no serious pathology exists. Patients should be well educated that hurt/pain does not mean harm, and pain does not mean damage. The clinician should repeatedly convey the message that exercise and keeping active are safe and effective. Once these pre-requisites are met, then graded activities can be introduced.

Evidence for functional rehabilitation programmes

An Italian study looked at functional rehabilitation for patients with fibromyalgia that was carried out over 10 sessions and a 5-week period. The study compared rehabilitation aimed at a specific tactile and proprioceptive approach with that of physical exercise alone or with a control group. Perceptual and physical exercise approaches both showed statistically significant improvements in outcome scores.

Research encompassing a fibromyalgia rehabilitation programme from Ontario, Canada, which was designed with 36 sessions over 12 weeks, concluded that the programme was effective in improving physical impairments and function.

A United States study on an 8-week functional rehabilitation programme demonstrated improved function and decreased disability in patients with fibromyalgia. The authors recommended that rehabilitation programmes should focus on function rather than on the pain.

Predictors of outcomes

The IMPROvE study (Interdisciplinary Rehabilitation and Evaluation Programme for Patients With Chronic Widespread Pain: Randomized Controlled Trial) looked at interdisciplinary rehabilitation for patients with fibromyalgia, with outcomes focusing on activities of daily living and assessment of motor and process skills 6 months after the programme. A meaningful improvement in motor and process skills was found in 38.7% of patients at 6 months post-intervention. The best predictors of recovery described in this study were found for patients who had a low baseline intake of analgesics and who had more pronounced clinical signs of central sensitisation.

Adherence to functional rehabilitation programmes

Functional rehabilitation is not always successful. Despite careful selection of patients in a musculoskeletal functional restoration programme, a 1-year prospective study showed that 21% of patients failed to complete the programme. Those who could not complete the programme were found to have worse levels of pain and impairment over the long term. Non-completers had lower socioeconomic outcomes and higher health utilisation outcomes in the long term.

Key Points

- Functional rehabilitation helps patients to return to their maximum possible level of independence in the activities that are important to them.
- The goals vary depending on the priorities and abilities of the patient.
- The evidence has shown an improved outcome both physically and functionally with these programmes.

References

1.   Costa ID, Gamundí A, Miranda JGV, *et al.* Altered functional performance in patients with fibromyalgia. *Front Hum Neurosci* 2017; 11: 14.

2.   Schofferman J. Restoration of function: the missing link in pain medicine? *Pain Med* 2006; 7 Suppl 1: S159-65.

3.   Paolucci T, Baldari C, Di Franco M, *et al.* A new rehabilitation tool in fibromyalgia: the effects of perceptive rehabilitation on pain and function in a clinical randomized controlled trial. *Evid Based Complement Alternat Med* 2016; 2016: Article ID 7574589.

4.   Bailey A, Starr L, Alderson M, Moreland J. A comparative evaluation of a fibromyalgia rehabilitation program. *Arthritis Care Res* 1999; 12(5): 336-40.

5.   Wennemer HK, Borg-Stein J, Gomba L, *et al.* Functionally oriented rehabilitation program for patients with fibromyalgia: preliminary results. *Am J Phys Med Rehabil* 2006; 85(8): 659-66.

6.   Amris K, Luta G, Christensen R, *et al.* Predictors of improvement in observed functional ability in patients with fibromyalgia as an outcome of rehabilitation. *J Rehabil Med* 2016; 48(1): 65-71.

7.   Proctor TJ, Mayer TG, Theodore B, Gatchel RJ. Failure to complete a functional restoration program for chronic musculoskeletal disorders: a prospective 1-year outcome study. *Arch Phys Med Rehabil* 2005; 86(8): 1509-15.

Chapter 28

Graded exercise therapy

Introduction

There have been significant controversies with regards to graded exercise therapy (GET) in chronic fatigue syndrome. As there is a significant overlap between chronic fatigue syndrome and fibromyalgia syndrome, this chapter will introduce the controversies surrounding GET for these conditions.

Graded exercise therapy

Graded exercise therapy (GET) is a programme that establishes an individual's baseline of achievable exercise or physical activity, and then makes fixed incremental increases in the time spent in these activities.

GET is usually delivered by physiotherapists with a gradual increase in aerobic exercises on a fixed time limit goal. After a careful assessment, an initial exercise duration is usually set between 5 and 15 minutes, which is increased slowly to 30 minutes for 4–5 days per week. Various protocols exist and one example would be to set a target heart rate of 40% of maximal oxygen consumption that is increased gradually to 60%. Patients who are averse to cognitive behaviour-based pain management models might find it easier to accept the GET pathway.

Evidence for GET

The PACE (Pacing, graded Activity, and Cognitive behaviour therapy; a randomised Evaluation) trial compared four different pathways in chronic fatigue: adaptive pacing therapy (APT), cognitive behaviour therapy (CBT), GET and specialist medical care. It found that CBT and GET are safe and effective ways to moderately improve outcomes, but APT was ineffective. The number needed to treat (NNT) for recovery with CBT and GET was quoted as seven by the authors of this trial, which was similar to that of the pharmacological agents used in this condition.

Another UK study followed this programme to look at recovery rather than effectiveness alone and concluded that GET and CBT were more effective than specialist medical care or APT. A 22% recovery was measured after CBT and GET participation, whilst it was only 8% after APT and 7% after standard specialist care.

A Belgian meta-analysis of GET in fibromyalgia recommended that it should be a part of a multidisciplinary programme, as most authors reported a benefit; however, the unequivocal benefit has not been established.

National Institute for Health and Care Excellence (NICE) guidelines and controversies

NICE guidelines clearly explain that there is no 'one size fits all' approach to managing symptoms in myalgic encephalomyelitis (ME)/chronic fatigue syndrome (CFS). There were controversies related to the role of GET when NICE published their guidelines; these forced NICE to release a statement in November 2020. NICE stated that due to the harm reported by people with ME/CFS, as well as the NICE Committee's own research of the effects when people exceed their energy limits, it did not recommend fixed incremental increases in exercise via GET for these patients.

This statement was completely different from the NICE recommendation in 2007 for CFS. This previous guidance concluded that CBT and GET should be offered to people with mild or moderate CFS or ME.

Limitation of GET

GET focuses on the physiological process of deconditioning and sensitisation and aims to improve these outcomes rather than looking at the cognitive behavioural pathway. It is time limited, in that graded exercises are increased over a fixed duration rather than focusing on the flare-up of pain that can occur.

A review quoted that symptom exacerbations from vigorous exercise/activity in GET can promote immune dysfunction, thereby increasing the symptoms of chronic fatigue. However, it recommended ways to gradually perform the exercise that avoided these side effects on the immune system.

A recent meta-analysis of ten trials including 1279 patients found that there was no evidence of excess harm with GET by either self-rated deterioration or by withdrawing from GET. However, this research documented that more GET participants dropped out on follow-up compared with the control group.

Flare-ups and relapse

Critics of GET have mentioned that the flare-up of pain and fatigue in fibromyalgia can be worse and, if it occurs, it can be a hindrance to the recovery pathway. The time taken to return to the physical activity level the patient had before taking part in GET can vary significantly between patients.

Individualised approach or fixed graded approach?

Patients with fibromyalgia have argued against the fixed graded approach. Some patients even lacked the energy to get out of bed, let alone being assessed for baseline energy for physical activities. These patients argued that the approach should be individualised, specific to that patient and their pain/fatigue level, rather than a fixed graded approach. Meticulous assessment and monitoring are essential to look for early signs of a flare-up of pain, fatigue or other symptoms. It is recommended that immediate attention is given and correction is implemented to manage the pathway.

Key Points

- GET establishes the individual's baseline of activities and then makes fixed increments in time spent on these activities.
- GET has a fixed time limit goal; critics argue that consideration should be made for a flare-up of pain.
- Controversies have prevailed over the NICE guidelines for GET; the recent guidelines do not recommend GET in chronic fatigue syndrome.
- Symptom exacerbation due to GET can be linked to immune dysregulation.
- An individualised approach with careful assessment of baseline and meticulous monitoring looking for a flare-up with immediate correction is recommended.

References

1. Moss-Morris R, Deary V, Castell B. Chronic fatigue syndrome. *Handb Clin Neurol* 2013; 110: 303-14.

2. White PD, Goldsmith KA, Johnson AL, *et al*. Comparison of adaptive pacing therapy, cognitive behaviour therapy, graded exercise therapy, and specialist medical care for chronic fatigue syndrome (PACE): a randomised trial. *Lancet* 2011; 377(9768): 823-36.

3. White PD, Goldsmith K, Johnson AL, *et al*. Recovery from chronic fatigue syndrome after treatments given in the PACE trial. *Psychol Med* 2013; 43(10): 2227-35.

4. Maquet D, Demoulin C, Croisier JL, Crielaard JM. Benefits of physical training in fibromyalgia and related syndromes. *Ann Readapt Med Phys* 2007; 50(6): 363-8.

5. National Institute for Health and Care Excellence. NICE draft guidance addresses the continuing debate about the best approach to the diagnosis and management of ME/CFS. Available from: https://www.nice.org.uk/news/article/nice-draft-guidance-addresses-the-continuing-debate-about-the-best-approach-to-the-diagnosis-and-management-of-me-cfs.

6. National Institute for Health and Care Excellence; 2007. Chronic fatigue syndrome/myalgic encephalomyelitis (or encephalopathy): diagnosis and management. NICE clinical guideline, CG53. Available from: https://www.nice.org.uk/guidance/cg53.

7. National Institute for Health and Care Excellence; 2021. Myalgic encephalomyelitis (or encephalopathy)/chronic fatigue syndrome: diagnosis and management. NICE guideline, NG206. Available from: https://www.nice.org.uk/guidance/ng206/chapter/Recommendations# managing-mecfs.

8. White PD, Etherington J. Adverse outcomes in trials of graded exercise therapy for adult patients with chronic fatigue syndrome. *J Psychosom Res* 2021; 147: 110533.

9. Nijs J, Paul L, Wallman K. Chronic fatigue syndrome: an approach combining self-management with graded exercise to avoid exacerbations. *J Rehabil Med* 2008; 40(4): 241-7.

Chapter 29

Breathing exercises

Introduction

Breathing exercises can reduce the levels of sympathetic chemicals that play a main role in the transmission of pain signals and fatigue. As a result, they are an important part of the relaxation strategies used in the fibromyalgia recovery pathway.

Breathing problems and fibromyalgia

A study of 87 consecutive chronic primary patients with fibromyalgia in a university hospital found that 84% of patients had symptoms of dyspnoea, as measured by the World Health Organization (WHO) dyspnoea grade. The authors explained that this was not explained by cardiac or pulmonary causes, but may be due to diaphragmatic muscular insufficiency and physical inactivity.

Another study with polysomnography in patients with fibromyalgia showed that these patients have many sleep arousals with apnoea-hypopnoea episodes; desaturation in sleep was common, with half of the patient group having a nadir oxygen saturation less than 87%.

People with fibromyalgia were found to have increased pain, linked to taking quick, short breaths, compared with a control population. In this study, slow breathing reduced pain intensity and unpleasantness.

Effectiveness of breathing exercises

Breathing exercises have a direct link to the functioning of the autonomic nervous system and are a useful 'way in' to reduce the hyperarousal and stressed state. By increasing our awareness of breathing, a patient with fibromyalgia can reduce the level of stress, improve their sense of well-being, and bring an interconnectedness between their mind and body.

Evidence for breathing exercises

A randomised trial of breathing exercises versus a control group in women with fibromyalgia showed that they produced significant benefits in terms of pain threshold tolerance on tender points and this predicted improvement in functional capacity to perform daily life, pain and fatigue.

An 8-week intervention with breathing exercises in patients with fibromyalgia ameliorated the threshold for pain tolerance and enhanced sleep quality.

In a qualitative study on fibromyalgia flares in 40 patients who were surveyed on how they dealt with the flare-ups, 18.2% of these patients regularly used breathing exercises to deal with the flares. This was the third commonest technique in this survey, next only to medications and massage.

Basic pre-requisites

Sitting comfortably in a correct posture without any outside distractions is important. Breathing in through the nose and out through the mouth is advised. Noticing the body movements and allowing the thoughts to come and go in the mind in a mindful manner are vital.

Calm abdominal breathing

Calm or deep abdominal breathing helps towards conserving energy and requires less effort to aid breathing. The patient is asked to sit in a relaxed position on a chair, then put one hand on the chest and the other hand on the abdomen. The patient is then asked to breathe in slowly through the nose and to breathe out through the mouth in a relaxed manner. Controlled breathing moves the hand placed on the abdomen, rising with inspiration and falling with expiration. Patients are guided to make expiration twice as long as inspiration, or even longer depending on their pattern, symptoms and response. Combining controlled breathing with a mindfulness approach, by focusing on thoughts to release stress/tension and on breathing, will also help towards relaxation. Gentle, gradual movements help in this process.

Various apps, such as Breathe2Relax, are freely available online and can be signposted to patients.

Other breathing strategies

Pursed lip breathing
This technique involves the patient breathing in through the nose and breathing out gently through the mouth, with their lips pursed, such as blowing a candle or whistling. Here, expiration is longer than inspiration. This can be done during any physical activity, including walking.

Blow as you go
During an activity that requires physical exertion, for example, going up the stairs, the patient is asked to breathe in and then to breathe out 'as they go'.

Paced breathing
Pacing breathing with activity can be helpful. For example, when climbing stairs, the patient breathes in on making one step and breathes out on making the next step.

Biofeedback and breathing
A trial of biofeedback training in patients with fibromyalgia to manipulate heart rate variability by breathing at their resonant frequency twice daily was

studied; the study found that there was an improvement in mood, pain and functioning from the start until the 3-month follow-up.

Posture and breathlessness

Patients can adopt a position that will reduce the effort of breathing, which, in turn, will help reduce breathlessness, for example, supporting the arms, rather than gripping them. Some patients find that dropping their shoulders might help with their breathing. Leaning forward might reduce the work done by the upper body and therefore also help with breathlessness.

Practise before use

The main advice that a clinician should give to the patient with fibromyalgia is to practise many times before use; if a patient tries this for the first time whilst having a flare-up of pain, it will not help them, and they might lose confidence in this strategy. Appropriate education, demonstration, practise to check that it is done appropriately and practising at least 5–10 minutes twice a day are vital before using this strategy in flare-up scenarios. Having a relaxed posture and allowing thoughts to come and go without hindrance in a mindful manner will help when performing the breathing exercises.

Key Points

- Slow breathing can reduce pain intensity and improve mood.
- Calm abdominal breathing is a commonly practised technique in fibromyalgia.
- Posture and relaxation are vital in any breathing technique.
- It is important to practise many times in a relaxed manner before using the technique in situations of a flare-up of pain.

References

1.   Royal College of Paediatric and Child Health, Calvert S; July 2020. Breathing exercises – a bridge between body and mind. Available from: https://www.rcpch.ac.uk/news-events/news/breathing-exercises-bridge-between-body-mind.

2.   Caidahl K, Lurie M, Bake B, *et al.* Dyspnoea in chronic primary fibromyalgia. *J Intern Med* 1989; 2 26(4): 265-70.

3.   Shah MA, Feinberg S, Krishnan E. Sleep-disordered breathing among women with fibromyalgia syndrome. *J Clin Rheumatol* 2006; 12(6): 277-81.

4.   Zautra AJ, Fasman R, Davis MC, Craig ADB. The effects of slow breathing on affective responses to pain stimuli: an experimental study. *Pain* 2010; 149(1): 12-8.

5.   Tomas-Carus P, Branco JC, Raimundo A, *et al.* Breathing exercises must be a real and effective intervention to consider in women with fibromyalgia: a pilot randomized controlled trial. *J Altern Complement Med* 2018; 24(8): 825-32.

6.   Garrido M, Castaño MY, Biehl-Printes C, *et al.* Effects of a respiratory functional training program on pain and sleep quality in patients with fibromyalgia: a pilot study. *Complement Ther Clin Pract* 2017; 28: 116-21.

7.   Vincent A, Whipple MO, Rhudy LM. Fibromyalgia flares: a qualitative analysis. *Pain Med* 2016; 17(3): 463-8.

8.   Vasu T. Managing breathlessness. In: Vasu T. *Managing long COVID syndrome.* Shrewsbury, UK: tfm publishing Ltd; 2022: pp. 163-7.

9.   Breathe. 2Relax app. Available from: https://play.google.com/store/apps/details?id=org.t2health. breathe2relax&hl=en_GB&gl=US.

10. Hassett AL, Radvanski DC, Vaschillo EG, *et al.* A pilot study of the efficacy of heart rate variability (HRV) biofeedback in patients with fibromyalgia. *Appl Psychophysiol Biofeedback* 2007; 32(1): 1-10.

Chapter 30

Massage therapies

Introduction

Self-management is the goal for recovery in fibromyalgia syndrome. Many passive therapies such as massage, heat and cold therapies, aromatherapy, hydrotherapy, acupuncture, and a transcutaneous electrical nerve stimulation (TENS) machine are used after proper education as multimodal therapy. Patients should be clearly advised on the limitations of these therapies before use.

Massage therapy

Massage therapy can have both physical and psychological benefits in the recovery pathway of fibromyalgia syndrome. It offers the opportunity to educate patients on supported self-management principles as part of their rehabilitation pathway, whereby patients should be encouraged to take control of their own recovery with the use of 'passive' treatment. Scientific evidence has been equivocal in the use of massage therapy in fibromyalgia and proper evaluation of its efficacy is needed.

Massage therapy involves the physical manipulation of soft tissues of the body. The Swedish or classic massage technique is usually applied in Western countries. Therapists from the Indian subcontinent use a traditional ayurvedic massage with herbal oils that is particularly popular in Kerala and regions in Southern India. Other techniques include sports massage, deep tissue massage, clinical massage and Eastern techniques (such as shiatsu, thai and tuina).

Mechanism of action

Massage can release the muscle trigger points and modulate the neurotransmitters in the pain pathway. It can reduce muscle tension in fibromyalgia. Immunohistochemical studies have shown increased levels of collagen and inflammatory mediators in the connective tissue surrounding the muscle cells in patients with fibromyalgia; massage can help ease these factors to relieve stiffness and pain.

As in other mechanical adjuncts that are used in pain relief, massage acts via the gate-control theory by modulating the neural pathway at the spinal cord level. The tactile non-noxious Aβ-fibres can be stimulated to block the pain signals via the relatively slower Aδ- and C-fibres at the dorsal horn of the spinal cord.

A study looked at the variations in 24-hour urinary levels of corticotropin-releasing factor-like immunoreactivity (CRF-LI), considered as a biochemical marker of stress-related symptoms in fibromyalgia, during massage therapy. Therapies such as massage and guided relaxation were effective in reducing the urinary levels of CRF-LI and this correlated with the levels of pain and emotional reactions.

Massage improves heart rate variability by decreasing sympathetic tone and increasing parasympathetic tone. Joint flexibility has been found to improve with massage with the amelioration of muscle stiffness.

Massage can provide global relaxation, thereby helping sleep; this can help in generalised pain neuromodulation to improve quality of life. Massage can also improve circulation, especially regional muscle blood flow; it can lower heart rate and improve the autonomic balance by reduced sympathetic drive and increasing parasympathetic drive.

Evidence for massage therapy

A review of six randomised controlled trials and two single-arm studies concluded that there is moderate evidence for massage therapy in fibromyalgia; however, the review suggested that massage should be gradually increased from session to session and should be performed at least one or two times a week.

Another research study on connective tissue massage showed an effect on pain relief of 30% in 3 months, but after 6 months the pain was back to 90%; the long-term beneficial effects of massage can therefore be questioned due to this finding.

A systematic review of the dose-response relationship between soft tissue manual therapy and clinical outcomes in fibromyalgia did not find any consistent dose-response relationship. The review suggested that for future research trials there should be a standard dose of 45 minutes manual therapy done 3–5 times per week for 3–5 weeks (totalling 11 hours 15 minutes).

A study comparing massage with use of a TENS machine showed that massage was more effective for pain and mood scores; however, this was analysed during the study over 5 weeks and long-term outcomes were not measured. Another study carried out over more than 5 weeks of massage showed that patients had improved sleep and decreases in substance P levels compared with the effects of relaxation therapy. A randomised controlled trial of 74 patients with fibromyalgia given myofascial release massage therapy over 20 weeks found that it improved pain, anxiety, sleep, mood and quality of life at 1 month after the last treatment session, but only improved sleep after 6 months.

The recently revised recommendations of the European League Against Rheumatism (EULAR) do not recommend massage. EULAR looked at six reviews and one meta-analysis; it concluded that massage was not associated with significant improvement in pain. However, there were intention-to-treat studies with favourable and non-favourable outcomes, both with significant results. There was some evidence of a positive effect for massage of more than 5 weeks' duration, but EULAR considered these trials to be of low quality. The EULAR group concluded that there was weak evidence against massage (86% agreement from the EULAR Committee).

Comparison of different types of massage

A meta-analysis of ten trials investigating different types of massage used to relieve fibromyalgia looked at narrative analysis and suggested that:

- Myofascial release improves fatigue, stiffness and quality of life.
- Connective tissue massage improves mood and quality of life.
- Manual lymphatic drainage is better than connective tissue massage for stiffness, mood and quality of life.
- Shiatsu massage improves pain, fatigue, sleep and quality of life.
- Swedish massage does not improve outcomes.

The authors quoted moderate evidence for myofascial release in fibromyalgia, but the above statements were based on narrative analysis only.

A randomised controlled trial that compared manual lymph drainage therapy with connective tissue massage in women with fibromyalgia found benefits for pain, health status and quality of life scores in both groups; manual lymph drainage therapy was found to be more effective than connective tissue massage.

One study showed that stretching exercises were better than friction massage and were effective for pain relief, similarly to analgesics. Stretching exercise produced longer effects than friction massage. The limitation of the study was that it assessed only 4 weeks of therapy.

Massage with exercise

A study comparing two 6-week programmes of either exercise with connective tissue massage or exercise alone showed that both groups had improved pain, fatigue, sleep and quality of life; however, the addition of massage therapy was found to have superior results in improving pain, fatigue, sleep and role limitations due to physical health compared with exercise alone.

Regulations for massage therapists

Unfortunately, in many countries, there are no regulating authorities for massage therapists; the profession is self-regulated and not regulated by law. There are voluntary registers in many regions (such as the Professional Standards Authority accredited register in the UK), but it is the duty of the patient to check the credentials of the provider and analyse these before going to the treatment session.

Massage as part of the recovery plan

The evidence for massage therapies in fibromyalgia is equivocal. For a practising clinician, it can be challenging to manage a patient with complex fibromyalgia; it is vital to have as many tools as possible in their armamentarium to deal with these groups of patients. When suggesting massage, it is vital to check that it is carried out by a qualified therapist who realises the limitations and the need for multimodal strategies and engagement in self-management recovery pathways.

Key Points

- Massage therapies can help both physically and psychologically in patients with fibromyalgia syndrome.

- Massage can reduce muscle tension, alleviate trigger points and change the neuromodulation pathway of chronic pain.

- Evidence is equivocal but it is a useful tool in the armamentarium of the clinician dealing with complex patients with fibromyalgia.

- The EULAR revised guidelines do not recommend massage; it was concluded that there is weak evidence against the use of massage in fibromyalgia.

- Supported self-management should be the goal of patient recovery, even if 'passive' massage therapies are used in the multimodal rehabilitation pathway.

References

1. Vasu T. Massage and hot and cold therapies. In: Vasu T. *Managing long COVID syndrome.* Shrewsbury, UK: tfm publishing Ltd; 2022: pp. 213-6.

2. National Center for Complementary and Integrative Health. Massage therapy: what you need to know?; 2019. Available from: https://www.nccih.nih.gov/health/massage-therapy-what-you-need-to-know.

3. Liptan GL. Fascia: A missing link in our understanding of the pathology of fibromyalgia. *J Bodyw Mov Ther* 2010; 14(1): 3-12.

4. Lund I, Lundeberg T, Carleson J, *et al.* Corticotropin releasing factor in urine – a possible biochemical factor in fibromyalgia: responses to massage and guided relaxation. *Neurosci Lett* 2006; 403(1-2): 166-71.

5. Bazzichi L, Dini M, Rossi A, *et al.* A combination therapy of massage and stretching increases parasympathetic nervous activity and improves joint mobility in patients affected by fibromyalgia. *Health* 2010; 02(8): 919-26.

6. Kalichman L. Massage therapy for fibromyalgia symptoms. *Rheumatol Int* 2010; 30(9): 1151-7.

7. Brattberg G. Connective tissue massage in the treatment of fibromyalgia. *Eur J Pain* 1999; 3(3): 235-44.

8.   Sturman S, Killingback C. Is there a dose response relationship between soft tissue manual therapy and clinical outcomes in fibromyalgia? *J Bodyw Mov Ther* 2020; 24(3): 141-53.

9.   Sunshine W, Field TM, Quintino O, *et al*. Fibromyalgia benefits from massage therapy and transcutaneous electrical stimulation. *J Clin Rheumatol* 1996; 2(1): 18-22.

10.   Field T, Diego M, Cullen C, *et al*. Fibromyalgia pain and substance P decrease and sleep improves the massage therapy. *J Clin Rheumatol* 2002; 8(2): 72-6.

11.   Castro-Sánchez AM, Matarán-Peñarrocha GA, Granero-Molina J, *et al*. Benefits of massage-myofascial release therapy on pain, anxiety, quality of sleep, depression, and quality of life in patients with fibromyalgia. *Evid Based Complement Alternat Med* 2011; 2011: ID561753.

12.   Macfarlane GJ, Kronisch C, Dean LE, *et al*. EULAR revised recommendations for the management of fibromyalgia. *Ann Rheum Dis* 2017; 76(2): 318-28.

13.   Yuan SLK, Matsutani LA, Marques AP. Effectiveness of different styles of massage therapy in fibromyalgia: a systematic review and meta-analysis. *Man Ther* 2015; 20(2): 257-64.

14.   Ekici G, Bakar Y, Akbayrak T, Yuksel I. Comparison of manual lymph drainage therapy and connective tissue massage in women with fibromyalgia: a randomised controlled trial. *J Manipulative Physiol Ther* 2009; 32(2): 127-33.

15.   Amanollahi A, Naghizadeh J, Khatibi A, *et al*. Comparison of impacts of friction massage, stretching exercises and analgesics on pain relief in primary fibromyalgia syndrome: a randomized clinical trial. *Tehran Univ Med J* 2013; 70(10): 616-22.

16.   Toprak Celenay S, Anaforoglu Kulunkoglu B, Yasa ME, *et al*. A comparison of the effects of exercises plus connective tissue massage to exercises alone in women with fibromyalgia syndrome: a randomized controlled trial. *Rheumatol Int* 2017; 37(11): 1799-806.

Fibromyalgia

Chapter 31

Heat and cold therapies

Introduction

Heat and cold therapies are commonly used in many chronic pain conditions; the evidence for their use in fibromyalgia syndrome is equivocal. If used safely, the number needed to harm (NNH) could be low and these are cheap physical modalities for use in fibromyalgia.

Heat therapy

Heat therapy, or thermotherapy, involves the application of heat in various forms, such as hot water bottles, heat pads, ultrasound, wheat bags and electric heating pads, to help relieve pain and fatigue. These are commonly used by many patients, although scientific evidence on their efficacy is limited.

Heat increases the blood supply, whilst reducing inflammation and oedema, and can reduce stiffness and muscle spasms. Theoretically, improved blood circulation and consequently oxygen delivery, can improve and speed up the healing process.

Mechanism of heat therapy

A mechanism-based approach predicted that stress acts both centrally and peripherally to cause sympathetic vasoconstriction and reduced endothelium-dependent vasodilation; this leads to painful muscular ischaemia. Chronic stress has also been found to cause mitochondrial damage and reduce blood flow. The application of heat can help to relieve peripheral vasoconstriction and can help in fibromyalgia syndrome. Sauna therapy with heat at 60°C for 15 minutes has been found to improve the endothelial function in blood vessels.

Studies have also proposed that heat can work in various other mechanisms: accelerating biochemical metabolic processes, reducing muscle tone, altering cellular immune modulation and increasing nerve conduction velocity.

The application of heat in healthy volunteers showed an increase in serum cortisol, plasma norepinephrine and epinephrine concentrations; heat also altered the composition of mononuclear cells in the blood due to elevated stress hormone levels. The study stated that this can increase serum β-endorphins and decrease substance P levels.

The gate-control theory of pain physiology is commonly quoted, although this explanation is oversimplistic when describing the mechanism of action of heat. Non-painful stimuli can open the gate and close the pain transmission fibres at the dorsal horn level of the spinal cord (please refer to Chapter 34 for more details).

Ways of applying heat therapy

Heat therapy can be applied superficially (heat pads, hot pack, etc.) or deeply (ultrasound, whirlpool bath, etc.). Some common ways that patients with fibromyalgia use heat therapy include:

- Heat pads or bags.
- Soaking a towel in hot water and applying it over painful areas.
- Hot water bath or warm shower.

- Heating pads that are electrically activated.
- Mud baths, steam baths, sauna.
- Mineral water baths.
- Whirlpool baths.
- Infrared therapy.
- Ultrasound therapy.
- Paraffin waxing.

Evidence for heat therapy

A study using near-infrared whole-body hyperthermia, delivering heat up to 38.1°C body core temperature followed by a 15-minute heat retention period as an adjunct, was compared with standard multimodal rehabilitation alone in patients with fibromyalgia; there were significant differences with improvement in affective and sensory pain with heat in post-intervention, at 3 and 6 months post-intervention. Secondary analyses showed an improvement in pain intensity, quality of life and tender point assessment. Moderate effect sizes were observed for all outcome measures. A recent meta-analysis of infrared radiation on various conditions, including four studies on fibromyalgia, concluded that infrared radiation decreased pain levels and decreased Fibromyalgia Impact Questionnaire (FIQ) scores for patients with fibromyalgia.

A systematic review of 11 studies with physical modalities in patients with fibromyalgia showed that thermal therapy reduced pain visual analogue scores (VAS), tender points and FIQ scores. The study also analysed other physical modalities including low-level laser therapy, electromagnetic therapy and transcutaneous electrical nerve stimulation (TENS), but concluded that thermal therapy was a more effective physical modality for fibromyalgia.

An inpatient multidisciplinary treatment with the addition of hyperthermia for severely progressive fibromyalgia syndrome showed a statistically significant improvement in functional capacity and fibromyalgia symptoms when patients were discharged from the hospital.

Use of heat therapies in practice

A German population survey showed that the prevalence of chronic pain lasting longer than 1 year was 39.5%; among this population, mud pack and heat treatment was the most popular treatment, along with oral medications, massage and exercises. The survey showed that two-thirds of patients used more than one type of these treatments.

Another survey of consumers consisting of patients with fibromyalgia showed that whole-body warmth therapy and thermal bathing were the top two effective management strategies; heat therapies ranked in four out of the top ten strategies in this consumer survey of patients with fibromyalgia.

A similar survey was carried out in the USA by the National Fibromyalgia Association (NFA) among 2569 patients with fibromyalgia. The survey showed that heat therapies were in the top three commonly used interventions and also ranked as one of the top three effective interventions.

Heat-based therapies can offer psychological benefits by improving mental well-being, enhancing relaxation and improving sleep. The use of heat therapy is cheap, convenient and widely accessible.

Moist heat might give skin better protection than dry heat; water has better heat conductivity than air and can prevent moisture from being removed from the skin.

Limitations of heat therapy

Awareness of skin hygiene is essential in heat therapy to prevent skin damage or burns. However, heat therapy is generally a harmless technique, so its careful application can be trialled on patients with fibromyalgia syndrome. Many rehabilitation programmes and pain/physiotherapy services use this approach as a part of the multimodal recovery pathway.

Cold therapy

Cold therapy can be suitable for some patients. Cold temperatures slow blood flow and can reduce swelling and pain.

Application techniques for cold therapy

Cold therapy can be applied in various ways:

- Ice application.
- Ice bag or cold pack.
- Bag of frozen vegetables applied over the area.
- Towel soaked in cold water.
- Ice bath.
- Ice massage.
- Cryotherapy.
- Cold showers.

Mechanism of action of cold therapy

Cold temperatures can reduce blood supply and therefore reduce swelling and pain in some patients. Cold can have an anti-inflammatory action because of this mechanism. Cold can increase the levels of plasma antioxidants and improve immune function. It can also affect the nerve conduction pathway.

Various proposals that cold therapy increases the immune system in patients with fibromyalgia have not been proven; some have quoted the benefits of the increased sympathetic tone following an ice-cold shower. This statement is controversial as many patients with fibromyalgia can already have an elevated sympathetic response.

As mentioned previously for heat therapy, cold can close the gate in the spinal cord via the gate-control theory to neuromodulate pain physiology (see Chapter 34 for more details).

Cold therapy can improve mood and give a sense of satisfaction to patients with fibromyalgia who have engaged in physical modality intervention.

Evidence for cold therapy

The outcomes of whole-body cold therapy were much better than those of heat therapy in a crossover study in patients with fibromyalgia, but this study looked only at pain scores for a 2-hour period and a 24-hour period, rather than the long-term outcomes. However, another randomised controlled trial of 32 trials showed that there was no significant difference between a cold group and a heat group when evaluating pain and muscle soreness. This study showed that the beneficial effects of cold therapy were significant within 24 hours of application, but there were no obvious effects on pain after 24 hours.

A randomised study on whole-body cryotherapy in patients with fibromyalgia showed an improvement in the short term for pain scores and quality of life. However, this study looked only at 2-week and 4-week intervals and did not look at long-term outcomes.

Harms of cold therapy

Cold therapy is often considered non-harmful; however, a German consumer survey of patients with fibromyalgia looked at 1600 questionnaires that assessed various physical, pharmacological and other approaches and quoted the local cold therapy as second on the list of harmful management strategies. Local cold caused harm in 5.1% of their survey population and nearly 40% graded the severity as 'high harm'. Whole-body cold therapy came tenth in the ranking, affecting 4.2% of the survey population. These were the only two non-pharmacological approaches listed in the harmful strategies out of the top ten in the survey.

Contrary to this, a United States survey from NFA showed that cold was used by 30% of patients with fibromyalgia who were surveyed, and that they ranked it at 4.8 on an effectiveness score ranging between 0 and 10. This contrasted with a German survey in which only 10% of patients used cold therapy and had an effectiveness score of 4 out of 10.

Shock can lead to sequelae if cold is applied suddenly all over the body. A proper assessment of the patient with appropriate skills is essential. If applied locally, and with appropriate care, cold can be a good tool for some patients to manage fibromyalgia pain.

Key Points

- Heat and cold topical therapies are commonly used in many pain management services for fibromyalgia syndrome.
- The evidence is equivocal but the NNH is low, and these are safe, cheap options. The long-term benefits of heat and cold therapy are yet to be proven.
- Supported self-management should be the goal of patient recovery, even if 'passive' therapies are used in the multimodal rehabilitation pathway.

References

1. Vasu T. Massage and hot and cold therapies. In: Vasu T. *Managing long COVID syndrome*. Shrewsbury, UK: tfm publishing Ltd; 2022: pp. 213-6.

2. Vierck CJ. A mechanism-based approach to prevention of and therapy for fibromyalgia. *Pain Res Treat* 2012; 2012: ID951354.

3. Biro S, Masuda A, Kihara T, Tei C. Clinical implications of thermal therapy in lifestyle-related diseases. *Exp Biol Med (Maywood)* 2003; 228(10): 1245-9.

4. Kappel M, Stadeager C, Tvede N, *et al.* Effects of *in vivo* hyperthermia on natural killer cell activity, in vitro proliferative responses and blood mononuclear cell subpopulations. *Clin Exp Immunol* 1991; 84(1): 175-80.

5. Jeziorski K. Hyperthermia in rheumatic diseases. A promising approach? *Reumatologia* 2018; 56(5): 316-20.

6.   PainScale. Heat or cold therapy for fibromyalgia. Available from: https://www.painscale.com/article/heat-or-cold-therapy-for-fibromyalgia.

7.   Brockow T, Wagner A, Franke A, *et al*. A randomized controlled trial on the effectiveness of mild water-filtered infrared whole-body hyperthermia as an adjunct to a standard multimodal rehabilitation in the treatment of fibromyalgia. *Clin J Pain* 2007; 23(1): 67-75.

8.   Tsagkaris C, Papazoglou AS, Eleftheriades A, *et al*. Infrared radiation in the management of musculoskeletal conditions and chronic pain: a systematic review. *Eur J Investig Health Psychol Educ* 2022; 12(3): 334-43.

9.   Romeyke T, Scheuer HC, Stummer H. Fibromyalgia with severe forms of progression in a multidisciplinary therapy setting with emphasis on hyperthermia therapy – a prospective controlled study. *Clin Interv Aging* 2015; 10: 69-79.

10. Samborski W, Stratz T, Sobieska M, *et al*. Intraindividual comparison of whole body cold therapy and warm treatment with hot packs in generalized tendomyopathy. *Z Rheumatol* 1992; 51(1): 25-30.

11. Wang Y, Li S, Zhang Y, *et al*. Heat and cold therapy reduce pain in patients with delayed onset muscle soreness: a systematic review and meta-analysis of 32 randomized controlled trials. *Phys Ther Sport* 2021; 48: 177-87.

12. Honda Y, Sakamoto J, Hamaue Y, *et al*. Effects of physical-agent pain relief modalities for fibromyalgia patients: a systematic review and meta-analysis of randomized controlled trials. *Pain Res Manag* 2018; 2018: 2930632.

13. Chrubasik S, Junck H, Zappe HA, Stutzke O. A survey on pain complaints and health care utilization in a German population sample. *Eur J Anaesthesiol* 1998; 15(4): 397-408.

14. Häuser W, Jung E, Erbslöh-Möller B, *et al*. The German fibromyalgia consumer reports – a cross-sectional survey. *BMC Musculoskelet Disord* 2012; 13: 74.

15. Bennett RM, Jones J, Turk DC, *et al*. An internet survey of 2,596 people with fibromyalgia. *BMC Musculoskelet Disord* 2007; 8: 27.

16. Rivera J, Tercero MJ, Salas JS, *et al*. The effect of cryotherapy on fibromyalgia: a randomised clinical trial out in a cryosauna cabin. *Rheumatol Int* 2018; 38(12): 2243-50.

17. Macfarlane GJ, Kronisch C, Dean LE, *et al*. EULAR revised recommendations for the management of fibromyalgia. *Ann Rheum Dis* 2017; 76(2): 318-28.

Chapter 32

Hydrotherapy

Introduction

Hydrotherapy utilises the benefits of the physical properties of water such as buoyancy, hydrostatic pressure and viscosity, thereby engaging patients in a gradual recovery pathway. Hydrotherapy also helps to improve mental well-being, which, in turn, further stimulates the patient's participation in their treatment. However, patients with fibromyalgia syndrome can have co-existing cardiorespiratory symptoms or postural orthostatic intolerance that can lead to difficulties; proper assessment is needed to determine the suitability of hydrotherapy in these patients.

Practicalities of hydrotherapy

An internet survey of 2596 people among patients with fibromyalgia showed that 74% of the responders used heat modalities (warm water, hot packs) and 26% used pool therapy. Pool therapy scored high with an effectiveness score of 6.0 ± 3.0 on a scale of 0–10.

Hydrotherapy or aquatic therapy utilises the properties of warm water to facilitate movement and achieve recovery in patients with fibromyalgia. Hydrotherapy generally refers to exercises in the pool under proper assessment and monitoring.

The buoyancy of the water supports the body's weight and eases the performance of exercises compared with exercises done on land. The hydrostatic pressure of water on the body helps to improve the core strength if targeted exercises are done gradually. Increased temperature and hydrostatic pressure can help circulation and reduce oedema if any. Heat can thereby reduce muscle soreness and joint pain.

Hydrotherapy can help to ease muscle stiffness and spasms and improve movement. It can reduce the pressure on weight-bearing joints.

It is not usually necessary in most rehabilitation programmes to be able to swim; the patient needs to stand in water and do specific movements that include walking in the water, lifting their legs and stretching.

Hydrotherapy can come in different forms: pool therapy involves movement in a pool; balneotherapy is drinking or bathing in medicinal water (which can include mineral water from natural springs or could include natural gases); spa therapy is bathing in thermal or mineral water. Hammam therapy uses scrubbing and cleansing techniques with the medium of water and/or steam. Peloid therapy uses mud or clay for therapeutic purposes. Thalassotherapy is a special form of balneotherapy that uses seawater and the seaside climate. These interventions are becoming popular as part of 'health resort medicine'.

Mechanism of action

Hydrotherapy can benefit the patient in various ways:

- Physical: improved movements, improved circulation, reduced oedema.
- Chemical: reduced inflammatory mediators.
- Psychological: improved confidence, satisfying experience, encourages relaxation.
- Social: boosts confidence, social support if carried out in a group setting, enables the learning of new skills, aids quicker recovery.

A study evaluating balneotherapy for the treatment of fibromyalgia syndrome looked at the serum levels of inflammatory markers; it found that, after balneotherapy, there was a significant decrease in the levels of interleukin 1 (IL-1) and leukotriene B4 (LTB4), suggesting the influence of the treatment on inflammatory mediators.

Hydrotherapy has also been suggested to increase the plasma levels of beta-endorphins, explaining their analgesic effect in patients with fibromyalgia.

Unspecific effects of hydrotherapy could include a change in environment, social effects, placebo-related neuromodulation, and holiday scenery (spa therapy).

A 16-week programme on hydrotherapy in women with fibromyalgia showed that it improved postural control, pain and function; postural control was measured with eyes open or closed, with right or left tandem on a force platform.

Types of activities

Hydrotherapy can be individually goal-based or can be done in a group setting. In the UK, it is usually done in a group setting for relaxation, stretching and to improve core stability. Treatments can have specific goals including, but not limited to:

- Relaxation of the muscles.
- Gradual stretching.
- Core stability.
- Improving posture and balance.
- Improving endurance.
- Strengthening exercises.
- Music-enhanced movements.
- Aqua exercises.
- Functional rehabilitation.

Evidence for hydrotherapy

A systematic review of ten randomised controlled trials showed that hydrotherapy gave only a short-term benefit towards pain relief and health-related quality of life in patients with fibromyalgia; the moderate reduction in pain and improvement in quality of life was maintained at a follow-up of 14 weeks. The study showed no efficacy in medical and mud baths. It concluded that hydrotherapy is a safe treatment option with high acceptance by the patients and low side effects.

Another systematic review also showed positive outcomes for pain, health status and tender point count, recommending strong evidence for the use of hydrotherapy in fibromyalgia syndrome.

A recent meta-analysis showed moderate-to-strong evidence for a small reduction in pain with hydrotherapy and improvement in health-related quality of life at the end of the treatment with hydrotherapy; however, there was no effect on depressive symptoms and tender point count. The analysis also showed moderate evidence of a medium-to-large size reduction in pain and tender point count following balneotherapy in mineral/thermal water based on five studies.

A study of spa therapy in fibromyalgia found benefits that lasted for 6 months with regards to quality of life but lasted only 1 month for pain and tender point count; it concluded that spa therapy had both short- and long-term benefits in fibromyalgia.

A randomised trial looking at the relationship between aquatic physical training and aerobic functional capacity in patients with fibromyalgia showed that aquatic therapy should be performed continuously to improve clinical symptomatology. Cardiopulmonary exercise testing (CPET) showed an improvement in VO_2 (volume of oxygen consumption) and improved clinical symptoms, but there was no association between these two. After 16 weeks of the therapy, these variables were reduced to near baseline, suggesting that aquatic physical training should be performed continuously to improve clinical symptomatology and aerobic functional capacity.

The European League Against Rheumatism (EULAR) looked at four reviews and 1306 participants and noted consistency regarding the evidence for hydrotherapy and balneotherapy in fibromyalgia; it found no difference in superiority of one over the other. EULAR suggested that there is weak evidence to support the use of hydrotherapy/spa therapy in fibromyalgia syndrome.

Key Points

- Properties of water such as buoyancy, hydrostatic pressure and viscosity help to improve the recovery pathway in fibromyalgia syndrome.
- Pool therapy is commonly used and has high effectiveness as per patient surveys.
- The evidence varies for hydrotherapy techniques, but EULAR supports hydrotherapy, albeit with a weak level of evidence.

References

1. Bennett RM, Jones J, Turk DC, et al. An internet survey of 2,596 people with fibromyalgia. BMC Musculoskelet Disord 2007; 8: 27.

2. Ardiç F, Ozgen M, Aybek H, et al. Effects of balneotherapy on serum IL-1, PGE2 and LTB4 levels in fibromyalgia patients. Rheumatol Int 2007; 27(5): 441-6.

3. Trevisan DC, Avila MA, Driusso P, et al. Effects of hydrotherapy on postural control of women with fibromyalgia syndrome: a single arm study. MYOPAIN 2015; 23(3-4): 125-33.

4. Langhorst J, Musial F, Klose P, Häuser W. Efficacy of hydrotherapy in fibromyalgia syndrome – a clinical meta-analysis of randomized controlled clinical trials. Rheumatology (Oxford) 2009; 48(9): 1155-9.

5. McVeigh JG, McGaughey H, Hall M, Kane P. The effectiveness of hydrotherapy in the management of fibromyalgia syndrome: a systematic review. Rheumatol Int 2008; 29(2): 119-30.

6. Naumann J, Sadaghiani C. Therapeutic benefit of balneotherapy and hydrotherapy in the management of fibromyalgia syndrome: a qualitative systematic review and meta-analysis of randomized controlled trials. Arthritis Res Ther 2014; 16(4): R141.

7.   Dönmez A, Karagülle MZ, Tercan N, *et al.* Spa therapy in fibromyalgia: a randomised controlled clinic study. *Rheumatol Int* 2005; 26(2): 168-72.

8.   Andrade CP, Zamunér AR, Forti M, *et al.* Effects of aquatic training and detraining on women with fibromyalgia: controlled randomized clinical trial. *Eur J Phys Rehabil Med* 2019; 55(1): 79-88.

9.   Macfarlane GJ, Kronisch C, Dean LE, *et al.* EULAR revised recommendations for the management of fibromyalgia. *Ann Rheum Dis* 2017; 76(2): 318-28.

Section 6

Complementary therapies

Fibromyalgia

Chapter 33

Acupuncture

Introduction

Complementary therapies are not part of conventional medical care, but are used alongside it to aid the multimodal and comprehensive pain management plan. All these therapies should include education on chronic pain management strategies holistically. Complementary therapy is used alongside conventional medical treatments, whereas alternative medicine is used instead of conventional treatments.

Acupuncture is a commonly used complementary therapy in fibromyalgia and is popular among these patients. It has been given a lower number needed to harm (NNH) but its efficacy is debated among healthcare professionals.

The main challenges to the use of acupuncture in fibromyalgia syndrome include:

- To realise their limitations and understand that it is a part of a multimodal management strategy.
- To find the right healthcare practitioner who will administer acupuncture as part of the biopsychosocial model and has expertise in chronic pain management.

Acupuncture and pain relief

Acupuncture is a part of traditional Chinese medicine that involves inserting thin needles into the meridians in the body to help with different ailments. It is a part of the spectrum of alternative medicine that could be used as a complementary tool in other treatments. It is generally safe if performed under aseptic conditions by a trained person; it can be an important part of the multimodal management of chronic pain conditions if carried out with the appropriate expectations and patient education.

Needles are inserted at typical acupuncture points (qi) or meridians, although this placing has been debated. Chinese beliefs include the correction of imbalance between yin and yang energies by these needles to correct the ailments.

Electroacupuncture involves stimulating the acupuncture needles with electricity and is proposed to increase the efficacy of pain relief. Moxibustion is the practice of burning herbs or dried plant materials near the skin's surface at the acupuncture points.

A Cochrane review suggested that, although fibromyalgia is not a diagnosis in Chinese medicine, the spectrum of this disorder is similar to bi syndrome, which was described in Chinese medicine 2500 years ago. Bi syndrome is divided into a number of patterns based on pain characteristics that lead to management in traditional acupuncture practice in Chinese medical systems.

Mechanism of action

Various theories have been proposed for the mechanism of how acupuncture works:

- Neuromodulation of the pain pathway.
- Release of endorphins.
- Muscle relaxation.
- Activation of the descending inhibitory pathways.
- Reducing activation of the pain matrix in the brain.
- Dry needling and trigger point release.

- Reducing inflammation.
- Change in chemical mediators in the pain pathway.

Evidence in fibromyalgia

A review published in 2011 looked at 57 systematic reviews of acupuncture for pain relief and concluded that there is little truly convincing evidence that acupuncture effectively reduces pain. This review mentioned that acupuncture failed to be demonstrably effective for fibromyalgia, but it seemed effective for neck pain. However, it cautioned that serious adverse effects continued to be reported.

A Cochrane review published in 2013 suggested that one in five individuals with fibromyalgia had used acupuncture treatment within 2 years of diagnosis. The review concluded that there was low-to-moderate level evidence that acupuncture improved pain and stiffness in fibromyalgia compared with no treatment and standard therapy. It also concluded that electroacupuncture was better than manual acupuncture for pain, stiffness, global well-being, sleep and fatigue in fibromyalgia. The study found that the effect of acupuncture lasted up to 1 month and was not maintained at the 6-month follow-up.

A prospective randomised trial showed that acupuncture significantly improved pain, fatigue and anxiety in patients with fibromyalgia. However, another systematic review published in 2007 included five randomised trials. Three trials suggested short-lived positive benefits, whilst two trials were negative in results; the authors of the review did not recommend acupuncture for fibromyalgia.

A 2016 trial of acupuncture in primary care for fibromyalgia showed that acupuncture reduced pain intensity at 10 weeks and that the effects persisted at 1 year compared with sham acupuncture. A recent meta-analysis published in 2019 of 12 randomised trials showed that acupuncture was significantly better than sham acupuncture in relieving pain and improving the quality of life with low-to-moderate evidence in the short term in patients with fibromyalgia. In the long term, acupuncture was superior to that of sham acupuncture. This review concluded that acupuncture is an effective and safe treatment for patients with fibromyalgia.

The European League Against Rheumatism (EULAR) looked at eight reviews that included 16 trials and 1081 participants. One high-quality review demonstrated that acupuncture resulted in a 30% improvement in pain. EULAR also found that electroacupuncture was associated with improvements in pain and fatigue. EULAR concluded with support for acupuncture in fibromyalgia with weak evidence.

Cost-effectiveness

As the acupuncture industry is unregulated, financial constraints can become a problem in patients with fibromyalgia. Therefore, appropriate discussions regarding the costs and the effectiveness of the therapy should be made if applicable. It should be confirmed that the patient understands these issues before the treatment is started.

A systematic review published in 2012 on the economic evaluations of acupuncture as a treatment for chronic pain estimated the cost per quality-adjusted life year (QALY) as £2527 to £14,976 per QALY. This cost is typically below the threshold quoted by the National Institute for Health and Clinical Excellence (NICE) in the UK (estimated between £20,000 and £30,000). The review concluded that acupuncture is a cost-effective intervention in chronic pain and is below the typical willingness to pay threshold.

Problems with acupuncture

Western medicine uses acupuncture only after the clinical diagnosis has been made and when all other sinister causes have been ruled out. The timely referral to other specialists should not be missed due to delays from acupuncture.

There are two main categories of problems with acupuncture: problems related to mismatch of patient expectations and problems related to the procedure.

Problems related to patient expectations

Patients with fibromyalgia will already have gone through a 'revolving-door' phenomenon of seeing many specialists and having many investigations and interventions. Some individuals present with unrealistic expectations that cannot be matched by the acupuncture therapist. Patients should be educated on the realistic expectations of the results of acupuncture and the limitations. Acupuncture is not a cure for any chronic pain condition but is used as part of the management strategy. Even if it helps, it will not completely remove the pain. This must be explained honestly and empathetically to the patient. Furthermore, if it helps, it will give only short-term relief, and needs to be repeated.

Problems related to the procedure

In many circumstances acupuncture therapy is not regulated. It is the duty of the patient to find the correct qualified therapist who can offer this intervention in a biopsychosocial model.

Administering acupuncture under sterile precautions with a single-use needle is essential. Infection transmission and visceral damage have been reported, but these risks can be avoided with the appropriate care and adequate training.

Data from the National Reporting and Learning System (NRLS) database in the UK between 2009 and 2011 found 468 safety incidents, but 95% were categorised as low or no harm. Common adverse events include retained needles (31%), dizziness (30%), loss of consciousness (19%), falls (4%), bruising or soreness locally (2%) and pneumothorax (1%). The reviewers warned that miscategorisation and under-reporting might distort the overall picture from this database.

Key Points

- Complementary therapies are used alongside conventional medical treatments.
- Acupuncture is generally safe if done by a trained person under aseptic precautions.
- Various mechanisms have been proposed for acupuncture, including neuromodulation and the release of endorphins.
- The evidence for acupuncture in fibromyalgia varies; EULAR supports the process with weak evidence for acupuncture in fibromyalgia.
- Although generally safe, databases have reported harm due to acupuncture.

References

1. Vasu T. Complementary therapies. In: Vasu T, Balasubramanian S, Kodivalasa M, Ingle PM, Eds. *Chronic pain management*. Shrewsbury, UK: tfm publishing Ltd; 2021: pp. 175-8.

2. Deare JC, Zheng Z, Xue CCL, *et al.* Acupuncture for treating fibromyalgia. *Cochrane Database Syst Rev* 2013; 5(5): CD007070.

3. Ernst E, Lee MS, Choi TY. Acupuncture: does it alleviate pain and are there serious risks? A review of reviews. *Pain* 2011; 152(4): 755-64.

4. Martin DP, Sletten CD, Williams BA, Berger IH. Improvement in fibromyalgia symptoms with acupuncture: results of a randomized controlled trial. *Mayo Clin Proc* 2006; 81(6): 749-57.

5. Mayhew E, Ernst E. Acupuncture for fibromyalgia – a systematic review of randomized clinical trials. *Rheumatology (Oxford)* 2007; 46(5): 801-4.

6. Vas J, Santos-Rey K, Navarro-Pablo R, *et al.* Acupuncture for fibromyalgia in primary care: a randomised controlled trial. *Acupunct Med* 2016; 34(4): 257-66.

7. Zhang XC, Chen H, Xu WT, *et al.* Acupuncture therapy for fibromyalgia: a systematic review and meta-analysis of randomized controlled trials. *J Pain Res* 2019; 12: 527-42.

8. Macfarlane GJ, Kronisch C, Dean LE, *et al.* EULAR revised recommendations for the management of fibromyalgia. *Ann Rheum Dis* 2017; 76(2): 318-28.

9. Ambrósio EMM, Bloor K, MacPherson H. Costs and consequences of acupuncture as a treatment for chronic pain: a systematic review of economic evaluations conducted alongside randomised controlled trials. *Complement Ther Med* 2012; 20(5): 364-74.

10. Wheway J, Agbabiaka TB, Ernst E. Patient safety incidents from acupuncture treatments: a review of reports to the National Patient Safety Agency. *Int J Risk Saf Med* 2012; 24(3): 163-9.

Chapter 34

TENS machine

Introduction

Transcutaneous electrical nerve stimulation (TENS) is a commonly used intervention in many pain clinics as a complementary therapy. It is usually administered by a pain nurse or a physiotherapist in the chronic pain service. It is not a cure, but can be used as an adjunct to pain relief.

TENS machine

The TENS machine is a small battery-operated instrument that applies a mild electrical current via electrodes connected to the machine by leads. Various factors that can be altered in a typical TENS machine include intensity, frequency and pulse width. Different patterns of current stimulation can be used in some TENS machines. Conventional TENS machines use low amplitude and high frequency that produce a strong but painless sensation.

The TENS machine is cheap, safe and gives control to the patient, which will help in the recovery pathway for chronic pain in fibromyalgia.

Mechanism of action

The gate-control theory is proposed as one of the mechanisms of the TENS machine for pain neuromodulation. This theory suggests that there is a neurological gate at the level of the dorsal horn in the spinal cord that can be modulated by various input signals that can alter the pain pathway. Mechanical stimulation via the fast thick myelinated Aβ-fibres (vibration sensations) can block pain transmission through the slow thin unmyelinated fibres (painful sensations) in the spinal gate.

Some specific pathways mentioned in the mechanism of action of TENS machines include:

- Sensitisation of dorsal horn neurons.
- Elevated gamma-aminobutyric acid and glycine.
- Inhibition of glial cell activation.
- Changes in substance P levels.
- Release of endogenous opioids with an increase in endorphin levels.

Evidence for the use of TENS in fibromyalgia

Most studies on the TENS machine are inconclusive as they lack high quality and are biased. As in other adjuvant therapies in fibromyalgia, the evidence for TENS therapy also is equivocal.

A Cochrane review published in 2017 concluded that the evidence was insufficient to either support or refute the use of TENS in patients with fibromyalgia. In addition, the studies were found to be at high risk of bias, especially regarding sample size. This conclusion means that we cannot suggest or exclude the use of TENS in fibromyalgia syndrome.

Another 2018 systematic review looked at eight out of 62 studies and concluded that TENS effectively reduced pain in people with fibromyalgia; adding that TENS with therapeutic exercise programmes had a greater effect than exercise alone.

A randomised comparison of active TENS with placebo TENS and no TENS in patients with fibromyalgia concluded that there is a significant decrease in pain and fatigue with active TENS. This study also found that the pressure pain thresholds were significantly increased at the site of TENS and outside the site of TENS, therefore suggesting that TENS might restore central inhibition in primary fibromyalgia syndrome. The study concluded that TENS has short-term efficacy in relieving fibromyalgia symptoms whilst the stimulator is active.

A study published in 2020 showed that 4 weeks of TENS use resulted in a significant improvement in movement-evoked pain and fatigue compared with placebo. In addition, improvement of the Patients' Global Impression of Change (PGIC) was also higher in the TENS group.

Limitation of the TENS machine

Use of the TENS machine is usually avoided for patients with pacemakers or implanted defibrillators. It is relatively contraindicated in epileptic patients and should not be applied on broken skin.

TENS should not be applied at the front of the neck to avoid the vasovagal response and also at the front of the chest. It should be avoided over a tumour or malignancy to prevent stimulation of cell growth.

The need for more evidence

We need more evidence to suggest or exclude the use of TENS in fibromyalgia syndrome. However, it is cheap and safe and could be easily used in the self-management pathway of fibromyalgia recovery. Evidence suggests that TENS helps in movement-evoked pain, and it is wise to combine it with exercise therapy. It also has a role in reducing fatigue in patients with fibromyalgia.

Key Points

- TENS is used as a complementary therapy in fibromyalgia; it is safe, cheap and gives control to the patient to manage their pain.

- The gate-control theory suggests that thick myelinated fibres modulate the thin unmyelinated pain fibres; various other chemical changes in the pain neuromodulatory system have been documented with the use of a TENS machine.

- A Cochrane review concluded that there was insufficient evidence for a role for TENS in fibromyalgia.

- Other reviews have supported with weak evidence the use of TENS in fibromyalgia, especially in short-term use.

References

1. Johnson MI, Claydon LS, Herbison GP, *et al.* Transcutaneous electrical nerve stimulation (TENS) for fibromyalgia in adults. *Cochrane Database Syst Rev* 2017; 10: CD012172.

2. Megía García Á, Serrano-Muñoz D, Bravo-Esteban E, *et al.* Analgesic effects of transcutaneous electrical nerve stimulation (TENS) in patients with fibromyalgia: a systematic review. *Aten Primaria* 2019; 51(7): 406-15.

3. Dailey DL, Rakel BA, Vance CGT, *et al.* Transcutaneous electrical nerve stimulation reduces pain, fatigue, and hyperalgesia while restoring central inhibition in primary fibromyalgia. *Pain* 2013; 154(11): 2554-62.

4. Dailey DL, Vance CGT, Rakel BA, *et al.* A randomized controlled trial of TENS for movement-evoked pain in women with fibromyalgia. *Arthritis Rheumatol* 2020; 72(5): 824-36.

Chapter 35

Osteopathy and chiropractic

Introduction

People with fibromyalgia often go through a 'revolving-door' phenomenon of seeing many specialists and healthcare workers. Due to the frustration caused by the limitations of standard medical care, they start looking for alternative treatments to help manage their pain and fatigue. Osteopathy involves physically manipulating muscles, connective tissues and bones to help various ailments; it aims to improve the body's overall healing system. Chiropractic deals with spinal adjustment and uses techniques to facilitate optimal nerve transition. Both osteopaths and chiropractors use different approaches to manipulation and are trained differently. Although these are considered complementary therapies in some countries, they have been accredited and registered with appropriate training in other countries.

Osteopathy

Osteopaths use various techniques in fibromyalgia syndrome. Muscle energy techniques look at stretching and contracting muscles to restore somatic dysfunction. Counter-strain allows applying mild strain in the direction opposite to the reflex. Myofascial release involves palpation and releasing the myofascial tissues that are causing the contraction of muscles. High-velocity thrusts involve short, sharp movements to the spine.

Osteopathy massage techniques are proposed to help improve muscle flexibility and break down dense connective tissue. There are theories to suggest improved blood flow and lymphatic drainage due to manipulation. Reduction of spinal hyperexcitability can lead to pain neuromodulation to ease the symptoms of fibromyalgia.

The General Osteopathic Council regulates osteopaths in the UK. The USA offers a Doctor of Osteopathic Medicine training that is equivalent to that of physicians.

Rare serious side effects of osteopathy of the neck area have been reported in the literature.

Evidence for osteopathy

The evidence for osteopathy in fibromyalgia syndrome is debatable. The European League Against Rheumatism (EULAR) provided weak evidence against massage in patients with fibromyalgia. The EULAR concluded that massage was not associated with a significant improvement in pain. A subgroup analysis revealed a positive effect with massage of 5 weeks' duration or more, but this was based solely on low-quality trials.

A recent randomised controlled trial consisting of a 6-week trial of osteopathy in patients with fibromyalgia showed that it had no benefit over sham treatment for pain, fatigue, functioning and quality of life.

A recent systematic review of seven studies showed that the effect of manual therapy on fibromyalgia was inconclusive based on a very low-to-moderate quality of evidence. Out of all the manual therapies, the study concluded that only general osteopathic treatment gave clinically relevant pain improvement compared with the control group. Among the therapies, myofascial release was the most common modality used.

Another systematic review of nine trials showed that massage therapy with a duration of 5 weeks or more provided immediate beneficial effects on improving pain, anxiety and depression in patients with fibromyalgia.

A randomised trial of patients with fibromyalgia showed that osteopathic manipulative treatment was more efficacious in treating fibromyalgia than standard medical care. In this study, patients were randomised into four groups; patients in the manipulation group and in the combined manipulation and teaching group had better outcome scores than the moist heat group or the control group.

A retrospective study of the use of the myofascial release approach of osteopathic manipulative treatment in patients with fibromyalgia showed that 71% of patients reported functional improvement after 1 month; in this study, the improvement in quality and life and pain after 4 months was significant.

A study of connective tissue manipulation combined with ultrasound therapy (ultrasound and high-voltage galvanic stimulation) was carried out in patients with fibromyalgia. The prospective study involved 20 sessions and was followed up after 1 year. Results showed that pain intensity, functional outcome and improvements in non-restorative sleep were significantly better in the treatment group in patients with fibromyalgia.

Chiropractic

Chiropractic involves the manipulation of the spine and joints to facilitate optimal nerve transition. The majority of practitioners use the vertebral subluxation theory to propose corrections. In recent times, they have extended their repertoire to use other strategies including manipulation, exercise, other physical modalities and a cognitive behavioural approach.

In the UK, the chiropractic profession is regulated by the General Chiropractic Council; in the USA, accreditation is through the Council of Chiropractic Education. Similar councils are in place in Canada and Australia, and a joint model of accreditation is done internationally.

Evidence for chiropractic

There is no conclusive evidence for chiropractic except for low-to-moderate evidence in back pain.

The European League Against Rheumatism (EULAR) gave strong evidence against chiropractic in patients with fibromyalgia. It looked at 13 trials, but these studies were poor quality and lacked robust interpretable data. In total, 93% of the Committee agreed with strong evidence against chiropractic use in fibromyalgia.

A review of chiropractic practice in fibromyalgia was carried out by the General Chiropractic Council on chiropractic guidelines and practice parameters; this review showed moderate evidence for massage and muscle strength training, but only limited evidence for spinal manipulation.

Another systematic review of randomised clinical trials revealed that there was insufficient evidence to conclude that chiropractic is an effective treatment for fibromyalgia.

A randomised trial looked at the benefits of adding chiropractic to resistance training in patients with fibromyalgia. The effects after 16 weeks of either resistance training alone (with ten exercises performed two times per week) or in addition to chiropractic were studied. Results showed that resistance training improved strength, the impact of fibromyalgia and functionality domains. Furthermore, if the resistance training was combined with chiropractic, it improved adherence and dropout rates of the resistance training and facilitated greater improvements in the functionality domain.

Risks due to chiropractic

Care should be taken for ailments that cause joint instability, for example, rheumatoid arthritis.

A potential serious risk of cervical manipulation includes vertebrobasilar artery stroke, which is rare; this can be avoided by appropriate training and regulation with the accreditation of these professionals.

The need for accreditation and registration

The training and accreditation for osteopaths and chiropractors are variable in different countries. Given the harm that untrained practitioners can cause, it is vital that these procedures are regulated by appropriate training and registration.

Inconclusive evidence for osteopathy and chiropractic

Most of the studies for osteopathy and chiropractic found that the benefits of their use were inconclusive due to low-to-moderate levels of evidence. In addition, the effects of these manipulative treatments were usually studied in the short term rather than looking at long-term events. However, the touch-based approach with a therapeutic relationship between the therapist and the patient can provide a good rapport to treat this functional pain syndrome. Understanding the biopsychosocial model and using a psychological modulation approach can improve the outcome of any manipulative approach.

However, it should be noted that these are complementary therapies. Appropriate care should be taken to ensure that indirect risks of delayed or missed diagnoses are avoided by verifying the appropriate training of these therapists.

Key Points

- Osteopathy involves the physical manipulation of muscles, connective tissues and bones.
- The evidence for osteopathy is still inconclusive in fibromyalgia.
- Among various interventions in osteopathy, manipulative treatment was better in outcome in short-term studies.
- Chiropractic involves the manipulation of the spine and joints to facilitate optimal nerve transition.
- The evidence is limited but, if combined with exercise, chiropractic can improve adherence to the treatment.
- In fibromyalgia, the EULAR concluded that there was weak evidence against osteopathy and strong evidence against chiropractic.

References

1. NHS. Osteopathy – how it's performed? Available from: https://www.nhs.uk/conditions/osteopathy/ what-happens/.

2. Macfarlane GJ, Kronisch C, Dean LE, *et al*. EULAR revised recommendations for the management of fibromyalgia. *Ann Rheum Dis* 2017; 76(2): 318-28.

3. Coste J, Medkour T, Maigne JY, *et al*. Osteopathic medicine for fibromyalgia: a sham-controlled randomized clinical trial. *Ther Adv Musculoskelet Dis* 2021; 13: 1759720X211009017.

4. Schulze NB, Salemi MM, de Alencar GG, *et al*. Efficacy of manual therapy on pain, impact of disease, and quality of life in the treatment of fibromyalgia: a systematic review. *Pain Phys* 2020; 23(5): 461-76.

5. Li YH, Wang FY, Feng CQ, *et al*. Massage therapy for fibromyalgia: a systematic review and meta-analysis of randomized controlled trials. *PLoS ONE* 2014; 9(2): e89304.

6. Gamber RG, Shores JH, Russo DP, *et al*. Osteopathic manipulative treatment in conjunction with medication relieves pain associated with fibromyalgia syndrome: results of a randomized clinical pilot project. *J Am Osteopath Assoc* 2002; 102(6): 321-5.

7. Dal Farra FD, Chiesa A, Risio RG, *et al*. Fast improvements in functional status after osteopathic manipulative treatment based on myofascial release in patients with moderate or severe fibromyalgia: a retrospective study. *J Complement Integr Med* 2021. doi: 10.1515/jcim-2021-0139, PMID 34766483.

8. Citak-Karakaya I, Akbayrak T, Demirtürk F, *et al*. Short and long-term results of connective tissue manipulation and combined ultrasound therapy in patients with fibromyalgia. *J Manipulative Physiol Ther* 2006; 29(7): 524-8.

9. Schneider M, Vernon H, Ko G, *et al*. Chiropractic management of fibromyalgia syndrome: a systematic review of the literature. *J Manipulative Physiol Ther* 2009; 32(1): 25-40.

10. Ernst E. Chiropractic treatment for fibromyalgia: a systematic review. *Clin Rheumatol* 2009; 28(10): 1175-8.

11. Panton LB, Figueroa A, Kingsley JD, *et al*. Effects of resistance training and chiropractic treatment in women with fibromyalgia. *J Altern Complement Med* 2009; 15(3): 321-8.

Chapter 36

Aromatherapy

Introduction

Aromatherapy involves the use of aromatic oils to improve physical and psychological well-being holistically. Unfortunately, this use is not regulated in many countries, with subsequent doubts about the quality and safety of these essential oils.

Practicalities

Essential oils are obtained through mechanical distillation and are concentrated plant extracts that retain the natural smell and flavour of the source. The chemical composition varies within a plant species or from one plant to another.

Common aromatherapy oils include oils such as lavender, eucalyptus, chamomile, clove, geranium, jasmine, lemon, sandalwood, tea tree, nutmeg, ginger, thyme and rosemary.

Aromatherapy works through the sense of smell and skin absorption, depending on the use. Oils can be used via diffusers, inhalers, sprays, bathing salts, and candles, or as body oils or lotions, and in steam baths and clay masks.

Aromatherapy can help with relaxation strategies and improve sleep.

Evidence for aromatherapy

There is no evidence of high quality to support aromatherapy in fibromyalgia.

A 4-week study on topical lavender oil in patients with fibromyalgia showed significant benefit in quality-of-life improvement measured by Short-Form (SF)-36 scores.

A survey of consecutive patients with fibromyalgia seen in a tertiary pain clinic showed that 98% of patients used some form of complementary and integrative therapies. Of these, 39% expressed that they had used aromatherapy for fibromyalgia. This study compared similar findings in the same institute 14 years ago; aromatherapy use had dramatically increased from 14.9% in 2003 to 39% in the 2017 survey.

Risks of aromatherapy

Some essential oils or carriers can irritate the skin, especially if applied without any dilution. In addition, some oils can be phototoxic; some can be irritants for pets.

The National Institute of Environmental Health Sciences issued a warning that lavender oil and tea tree oil can lead to endocrine disruption with varying effects on the receptors for hormones, oestrogen and androgen.

Some essential oils can be toxic when taken internally. They should be kept out of the reach of small children due to these risks.

Sales of essential oils for medical purposes are not regulated in many countries; the quality and purity need to be checked and researched before use.

Key Points

- Aromatherapy uses essential oils to improve well-being.
- In most countries, the sale of essential oils for medical use is unregulated.
- There is no evidence for aromatherapy in fibromyalgia, but surveys show that it is used commonly by patients.

References

1. Yasa Ozturk GY, Bashan I. The effect of aromatherapy with lavender oil on the health-related quality of life in patients with fibromyalgia. *J Food Qual* 2021; 2021: ID9938630.

2. National Institute of Environmental Health Sciences. Lavender oil linked to early breast growth in girls; 2019. Available from: https://factor.niehs.nih.gov/2019/9/feature/3-feature-lavender/.

3. Mohabbat AB, Mahapatra S, Jenkins SM, *et al*. Use of complementary and integrative therapies by fibromyalgia patients: a 14-year follow-up study. *Mayo Clin Proc Innov Qual Outcomes* 2019; 3(4): 418-28.

Fibromyalgia

Chapter 37

Herbal remedies

Introduction

Herbal remedies are active ingredients extracted from plants to help with ailments. Botanical medicines can be derived from plant roots, leaves, stems, seeds, flowers or bark. Usually, these are not tested as for conventional medicines and are not regulated.

Practicalities

Herbal remedies are usually taken orally as extracts of plants; the infusion of these herbs in hot water or decoctions (boiled extracts) is also practised. A tincture is an alcoholic extract of the herb. Maceration is a cold infusion of a plant left to stand for a long time.

Safety issues

The consumption of untested herbs can lead to severe toxicity. Therefore, the quality of the herbal extract and its purity should be researched before use. The Committee on Herbal Medicinal Products regulates its use in Europe. The United States Food and Drug Administration (US FDA) regulates the use of dietary supplements in the USA; however, if they do not make medical claims, they do not need proof of safety or efficacy.

A review of herbal medicines in fibromyalgia showed various side effects, including transient burning and prickling, skin irritation, dizziness, nausea, dry mouth, drowsiness, constipation and insomnia.

Evidence for herbal remedies

Systematic reviews of herbal remedies in fibromyalgia are inconclusive and vary depending on the herbal extract used. Due to the heterogeneity of herbal remedies, it is difficult to analyse the evidence constructively.

A review of eight randomised placebo-controlled trials involving 475 patients concluded that medicinal plants or related natural products produced significant effects for improving the symptoms of fibromyalgia compared with conventional drugs or placebo.

Topical capsaicin from chilli pepper improved pain score, pressure pain threshold and global impact. A randomised study of 134 patients with fibromyalgia with topical 0.075% capsaicin administered three times a day for 6 weeks resulted in a significant improvement in the myalgic score and global subjective improvement compared with controls.

O24™ oil, which contains camphor, eucalyptus oil, aloe vera oil, peppermint oil, lemon and orange oil, has been studied for use in fibromyalgia with varying results. It has been proposed that this oil locally inhibits pain transmitters such as bradykinin, histamine and prostaglandins. Meta-050, containing magnesium salt of *Humulus* extract, rosemary and oleanolic acid, moderately improved pain and stiffness in fibromyalgia after 8 weeks.

Nabilone, made from cannabinoid extract, has shown positive results in fibromyalgia (further discussed in Chapter 47).

In a study using coenzyme Q10 and Ginkgo biloba extract in patients with fibromyalgia, 68% of participants who took this herbal remedy wanted to continue the treatment after 12 weeks. The majority (64%) felt that the treatment was of some benefit.

St. John's wort (*Hypericum perforatum*) has been suggested to help patients with fibromyalgia due to its antidepressant potential and serotonin modulation; this recommendation was only through narrative reviews rather than scientific evidence. One review quoted the risks of mood disorders and the caution needed to be taken to identify mania and hypomania.

Key Points

- Herbal remedies are usually not tested and are not regulated.
- Systematic reviews are inconclusive and do not allow recommending herbal treatments for fibromyalgia syndrome.
- Various herbal remedies have been tested for fibromyalgia, including capsaicin and nabilone, which are used in conventional medical systems.
- Risks and safety issues necessitate the rigorous testing and evaluation of herbal products.

References

1. de Souza Nascimento S, DeSantana JM, Nampo FK, *et al.* Efficacy and safety of medicinal plants or related natural products for fibromyalgia: a systematic review. *Evid Based Complement Alternat Med* 2013; 2013: 149468.

2. Casanueva B, Rodero B, Quintial C, *et al.* Short-term efficacy of topical capsaicin therapy in severely affected fibromyalgia patients. *Rheumatol Int* 2013; 33(10): 2665-70.

3. Perry R, Leach V, Davies P, *et al.* An overview of systematic reviews of complementary and alternative therapies for fibromyalgia using both AMSTAR and ROBIS as quality assessment tools. *Syst Rev* 2017; 6(1): 97.

4. Lister RE. An open, pilot study to evaluate the potential benefits of coenzyme Q10 combined with Ginkgo biloba extract in fibromyalgia syndrome. *J Int Med Res* 2002; 30(2): 195-9.

5. Kalcev G, Testa G, Manconi M, *et al. Hypericum scruglii Bacch., Brullo* & *Salmeri*, a potential natural remedy for fibromyalgia: a narrative review. *Biointerface Res Appl Chem* 2021; 11(3): 9928-38.

Fibromyalgia

Chapter 38

Hypnotism

Introduction

Hypnosis is a trance-like mental state induced carefully by a trained hypnotist to increase attention and suggestibility. Hypnosis can be used to neuromodulate the pain pathway in patients with fibromyalgia and increase movement and acceptance strategies. As in any other complementary therapy, it is very important to find a therapist who has had the correct training and possesses the relevant credentials before engaging in hypnosis therapy.

Mechanism of action

The pain neuromatrix theory proposes that, in chronic pain conditions such as fibromyalgia, there are changes in the network in the brain neuromatrix that lead to a persistent pain state. The neurosignature signals that make this neuromatrix can be altered by various factors, including genetic, environmental, changes in memory and experience, psychological status, the response from external factors and social factors. The neuromatrix continuously evolves based on input factors and the effect of various external responses. Hypnosis can be used to modulate this neuromatrix and the pain pathway.

The trauma theory considers significant past adverse life events as a causative factor in fibromyalgia; hypnosis can help the therapist uncover these past events and help in the patient's neuroprocessing and coping mechanisms. A study comparing hypnosis with clinical interviews showed that hypnosis was 9.8 times more effective in patients with fibromyalgia when expressing their traumatic life events than when awake during clinical interviews.

Neuromodulation and hypnosis

One study used a functional magnetic resonance imaging scan (fMRI) to look at differences between hypnotic induction and suggestion without hypnosis; both processes led to significant changes in the reported pain experience, but the effects were increased in hypnotised patients. Hypnotised patients claimed significantly more control over their pain. The areas activated in the fMRI scan were directly involved in the network of areas that have been widely associated with the pain 'neuromatrix' in fibromyalgia.

Another research study using a positron emission tomography (PET) scan to measure regional cerebral blood flow whilst using hypnosis in patients with fibromyalgia concluded a multifactorial nature of hypnotic analgesia, with an interplay between cortical and subcortical brain dynamics. In addition, patients had less pain during hypnosis than at rest.

Side effects and risks

Mild-to-moderate side effects include anxiety, dizziness, feeling tired and headache. Therefore, recovery from fibromyalgia should depend on providing the patient with self-management strategies to take control of their pain and fatigue; hypnosis might deviate from this pathway as the patient can become passively dependent on the therapist.

Evidence for hypnosis in fibromyalgia

Some studies have shown the benefit of hypnosis in fibromyalgia syndrome, but these were of low quality and insufficient size. Many studies combined hypnosis with other psychological strategies, making it difficult to distinguish the effects of hypnosis from other suggestive psychological modalities.

A systematic review of seven randomised controlled trials of patients with fibromyalgia showed a clinically relevant benefit of guided imagery/hypnosis compared with a control group with regard to ≥50% pain relief and psychological distress. In addition, two randomised trials showed that the combination of hypnosis and cognitive behavioural therapy (CBT) produced superior results compared with CBT alone in terms of psychological distress.

A randomised trial of five hypnosis sessions over 2 months in patients with fibromyalgia documented a significant improvement in the Patients' Global Impression of Change (PGIC) scale, sleep and the dramatisation subscale of the Cognitive Strategy Questionnaire.

A recent study investigating self-administered audio-recorded hypnosis in patients with fibromyalgia showed a reduction in intensity and interference of pain, fatigue and depression symptoms. These results suggested that audio-recorded clinical hypnosis was an effective, practical and cheaper alternative for the treatment of fibromyalgia.

Techniques in hypnosis

A randomised trial of patients with fibromyalgia looked at three test groups: hypnosis with analgesia suggestions, hypnosis with relaxation suggestions and relaxation alone. Outcomes were measured on a visual analogue scale and on the McGill pain questionnaire. The 'hypnosis with analgesia suggestions' group documented the greatest effect on pain and sensory dimensions of all three groups. However, the effect of hypnosis followed by relaxation was not greater than relaxation alone.

Self-hypnosis can be used in fibromyalgia with the appropriate training; it can enhance the efficacy of self-suggestion. It helps the patient to take control and be in charge of the suggestions. Trials of audio-recorded self-hypnosis showed a significant improvement in pain and fatigue levels, and these benefits were also sustained at the 6-month evaluation.

Key Points

- Hypnosis is a trance-like mental state used to increase attention and suggestibility.
- Hypnosis can neuromodulate and change the pain neuromatrix output in patients with fibromyalgia.
- Hypnosis increases the chances of patients expressing their past traumatic events.
- The evidence from scientific studies is not of high quality to support hypnosis in fibromyalgia.

References

1. Almeida-Marques FX, Sánchez-Blanco J, Cano-García FJ. Hypnosis is more effective than clinical interviews. *Int J Clin Exp Hypn* 2018; 66(1): 3-18.

2. Derbyshire SWG, Whalley MG, Oakley DA. Fibromyalgia pain and its modulation by hypnotic and non-hypnotic suggestion: an fMRI analysis. *Eur J Pain* 2009; 13(5): 542-50.

3. Wik G, Fischer H, Bragée B, et al. Functional anatomy of hypnotic analgesia: a PET study of patients with fibromyalgia. *Eur J Pain* 1999; 3(1): 7-12.

4. Zech N, Hansen E, Bernardy K, Häuser W. Efficacy, acceptability and safety of guided imagery/hypnosis in fibromyalgia – a systematic review and meta-analysis of randomized controlled trials. *Eur J Pain* 2017; 21(2): 217-27.

5. Picard P, Jusseaume C, Boutet M, et al. Hypnosis for management of fibromyalgia. *Int J Clin Exp Hypn* 2013; 61(1): 111-23.

6. Aravena V, García FE, Téllez A, Arias PR. Hypnotic intervention in people with fibromyalgia: a randomized controlled trial. *Am J Clin Hypn* 2020; 63(1): 49-61.

7. Castel A, Pérez M, Sala J, et al. Effect of hypnotic suggestion on fibromyalgic pain: comparison between hypnosis and relaxation. *Eur J Pain* 2007; 11(4): 463-8.

Chapter 39

Ayurveda therapy

Introduction

Ayurveda is an Indian natural system of medicine that has been practised for more than 3000 years. In the Sanskrit language, 'Ayur' means life, and 'Veda' refers to knowledge, meaning the knowledge of life or longevity. Ayurveda uses lifestyle interventions and natural therapies to regain control of the body with ailments. It involves diet, herbal remedies, yoga, meditation, massage and medical oils. Sushruta Samhita (600 BCE) and Charaka Samhita (200 BCE) are ancient Indian texts that provide evidence of ayurvedic practice on the Indian subcontinent.

In 2014, the Indian Government formed a Ministry of Ayush (Ayurveda, Yoga and naturopathy, Unani, Siddha, and Homeopathy) to educate, research and propagate indigenous and alternative medical systems.

Principles of Ayurveda

'Dosha' is the central tenet of Ayurveda that is assumed to cause imbalances in the body during ailments. These are of three types: vata (characterising movement, an important factor in pain conditions), pitta (representing metabolism and energy in the body), and kapha (representing nourishment and water component of the body). A trained practitioner can diagnose the imbalance of these three factors and will try to correct the imbalance with various strategies.

In the published literature, fibromyalgia is equated to snayugatavata in ayurvedic terms; fibromyalgia is considered an imbalance of vata dosha or termed as vata vyadhi (disease involving vata dosha).

Pranayama

Pranayama is the breathing technique used in yogic practice and is commonly practised in Ayurveda; 'prana' means 'vital life force' and 'yama' means 'control'. The three phases of breathing include inspiration (purak), plateau (kumbhak) and expiration (rechak). There is good evidence suggesting that breathing techniques can reduce sympathomimetic amines and thereby reduce stress and pain levels.

Meditation and mindfulness

Meditation is a common technique used in Ayurveda; it involves focusing the mind on a particular thought or object to improve attention and awareness, to calm and relax the practitioner. Most Indian techniques include pronouncing a mantra (group of syllables or words that are considered sacred), sitting in particular positions (asanas), using prayer beads or other religious techniques. In addition, mindfulness-based techniques that have been researched in Western practice are equivalent to the Indian and Buddhist systems of meditation.

Yoga

Yoga involves physical, mental and spiritual practices to control the mind with a detached feeling of mental and physical experiences. It has been practised ever since the time of Rig Veda, an ancient Indian script written in approximately 1500 BCE. It is practised widely in the Western world with an emphasis on posture, physical fitness and relaxation strategies. For example, a survey in 2012 estimated that 8.7% of the United States population practised yoga; it was estimated that 10.3 billion dollars were spent on yoga-related expenses. Another international survey of 2543 patients diagnosed with fibromyalgia showed that 79.8% had considered trying yoga, and 57.8% had attended at least one yoga class. The respondents cited the benefits of reduced stiffness, relaxation and better balance.

Modern yoga systems practise asanas, which involve gentle physical activities with smooth transitions combined with breathing exercises to aim for relaxation. One of the commonly practised exercises is the Surya Namaskar (sun salutation), which consists of the flow of a sequence of 12 graceful asanas.

An average metabolic equivalent energy expenditure is estimated to be approximately 3.3 metabolic equivalents of task (MET), equating to light-to-moderate aerobic intensity (3–6 MET) as classified by the American Heart Association. However, Surya Namaskar meets the criteria of moderate-to-vigorous intensity activity, as the average estimations of this exercise can vary from 2.9 to 7.4 MET, depending on the speed and experience of the performer.

Evidence for yoga

A systematic review of meditative movement therapies (qigong, tai chi and yoga) in fibromyalgia syndrome was conducted and the therapies compared. In general, these therapies reduced sleep disturbance, fatigue, depression and the limitations of a health-related quality of life (HRQoL), but there were no improvements in pain. These benefits were maintained after a median of 4.5 months as per the review. In a subgroup analysis, only yoga yielded significant effects on pain, fatigue, depression and HRQoL at the final treatment.

An 8-week study using yoga and meditation to manage fibromyalgia symptoms showed significant improvements in the patient report of the number of days they 'felt good'. However, pain and fatigue showed non-significant improvements.

Another 8-week 'yoga of awareness' programme for patients with fibromyalgia included 40 minutes of gentle stretching poses, 25 minutes of meditation, 10 minutes of breathing techniques, 20 minutes of coping education, and 25 minutes of group discussions. Compared with the control group, the yoga group showed significant improvements in symptom measures, pain levels, fatigue and mood.

Herbal remedies

The majority of the medications used in Ayurveda are from plants.

Commonly used herbs in Ayurveda that are used in various symptoms of fibromyalgia syndrome include:

- Turmeric (curcumin): considered anti-inflammatory; also sold and used commonly in the Western world. It should not be used in some vata conditions and can cause constipation.
- Tulsi (*Ocimum sanctum*): considered a holy plant, leaves can be eaten raw and considered to improve immunity.
- Indian gooseberry (nellikai or amalaki): improves the digestive system and nourishment, is liver protective and modulates oxidative stress and the immune response. It contains high levels of vitamin C.
- Ginger: useful for gastrointestinal problems.
- Aloe vera: used in many products for skin problems and can be anti-inflammatory.
- Pippali (thippali): can improve immunomodulation.
- Moringa (drumstick): commonly used as a vegetable.

A few commonly used herbal medications in Ayurveda include:

- Triphala: extracts from three fruits (haritaki, bibhitaki and amalaki); it is assumed to remove toxins from the body by opening channels in the body.
- Ashwagandha (*Withania somnifera*): extracts from the roots affect the central nervous system and can possess hypnotic, sedative and analgesic effects. It contains the alkaloid somniferin.

Opioids and cannabinoids are also used in Ayurveda as per the records. Moreover, Ayurveda also contains various surgical expertise as per the treatises.

Evidence for Ayurveda

Ayurveda has been practised for more than 3000 years on the Indian subcontinent, but Western scientific evidence is lacking due to a lack of high-quality studies.

A 2-year follow-up study of patients with fibromyalgia in an ayurvedic centre in Norway using a Fibromyalgia Impact Questionnaire (FIQ) showed that there were significant reductions (26% to 44%) in six of the seven dimensions: working ability, pain, tiredness, morning tiredness, stiffness and anxiety. The seventh dimension of depression was reduced by 32% and was borderline significant. This centre used transcendental meditation, panchakarma therapy, herbal products and diet changes.

A 2-week study of additive complex ayurvedic treatment in patients with fibromyalgia was compared with conventional standard care alone in a tertiary specialist rheumatology hospital in Germany. Although the study concluded that ayurvedic therapy was non-inferior to conventional treatment regarding improvement in FIQ scores, Ayurveda was only an add-on treatment in this study rather than a stand-alone therapy.

Caution and side effects

Unfortunately, many herbal products used in Ayurveda can have significant side effects and should only be taken under the supervision of a trained practitioner. In addition, some of these medications can react with other Western medications, especially anticoagulants and anti-inflammatory medications, potentiating their effects.

Some advertised ayurvedic medicines contain heavy metals that can be toxic to humans. For example, a publication from the USA found a substantial proportion of lead, mercury and arsenic in traditional ayurvedic medications manufactured in India and sold on the internet. However, Rasa Shastra is a subspeciality of Ayurveda in which metals, minerals or gems in very small precise quantities are deliberately combined with herbs to achieve the proposed benefits in certain ailments.

The ayurvedic market is unregulated, with many untested products; many can vary in content quality and dose as they are not standardised. Care and research are essential before use and it is vital to consult a qualified practitioner before administration.

Key Points

- Ayurveda is an Indian natural system of medicine that has been practised for more than 3000 years.
- It considers ailments as imbalances in three dosha systems: vata, pitta and kapha.
- Breathing strategies, meditation, yoga and herbal remedies are part of the ayurvedic therapy.
- Yoga is extensively practised in the Western world and has been trialled in the treatment of fibromyalgia.
- There is some evidence for the benefits of yoga in patients with fibromyalgia, but high-quality systematic reviews are still forthcoming.
- Herbal remedies are commonly used in Ayurveda; triphala and ashwagandha have been trialled in fibromyalgia.
- Herbal remedies can have side effects and need to be researched carefully before use.
- Studies have shown a benefit on scores of FIQ following Ayurveda treatment.

References

1. Shettigar DSS, Patil DUA, Prasad DS. A comparative clinical study on the efficacy of siravyadha and agnikarma in the management of snayugata vata affecting kurpara sandhi vis-à-vis tennis elbow. *JAIMS* 2018; 3(4): 14-7.

2. Yoga Journal. New study finds more than 20 million yogis in U.S. 2012.

3. Firestone KA, Carson JW, Mist SD, *et al.* Interest in yoga among fibromyalgia patients: an international internet survey. *Int J Yoga Therap* 2014; 24: 117-24.

4. Larson-Meyer DE. A systematic review of the energy cost and metabolic intensity of yoga. *Med Sci Sports Exerc* 2016; 48(8): 1558-69.

5. Langhorst J, Klose P, Dobos GJ, *et al.* Efficacy and safety of meditative movement therapies in fibromyalgia syndrome: a systematic review and meta-analysis of randomized controlled trials. *Rheumatol Int* 2013; 33(1): 193-207.

6. Hennard J. A protocol and pilot study for managing fibromyalgia with yoga and meditation. *Int J Yoga Therap* 2011; 21(21): 109-21.

7. Carson JW, Carson KM, Jones KD, *et al.* A pilot randomized controlled trial of the yoga of awareness program in the management of fibromyalgia. *Pain* 2010; 151(2): 530-9.

8. Kumar S, Dobos GJ, Rampp T. The significance of ayurvedic medicinal plants. *J Evid Based Complementary Altern Med* 2017; 22(3): 494-501.

9. Saper RB, Phillips RS, Sehgal A, *et al.* Lead, mercury, and arsenic in US- and Indian-manufactured ayurvedic medicines sold via the internet. *JAMA* 2008; 300(8): 915-23.

10. Rasmussen LB, Mikkelsen K, Haugen M, *et al.* Treatment of fibromyalgia at the Maharishi Ayurveda health centre in Norway II – a 24-month follow-up pilot study. *Clin Rheumatol* 2012; 31(5): 821-7.

11. Kessler CS, Ostermann T, Meier L, *et al.* Additive complex ayurvedic treatment in patients with fibromyalgia syndrome compared to conventional standard care alone: a nonrandomized controlled clinical pilot study (KAFA trial). *Evid Based Complement Alternat Med* 2013; 2013: 751403.

Fibromyalgia

Chapter 40

Siddha therapy

Introduction

The Siddha system of medicine originated from Tamil Nadu, a state in southern India. It is one of the earliest traditional systems of medicine in the world, dating back to 2000 BCE. Siddha originates from the word 'Siddhi', meaning 'heavenly bliss' in the Tamil language. This medical system treats people as a whole, examining the affected person's physical, psychological, social and spiritual well-being.

The Siddha system believes that the five basic elements — earth, air, sky, water and fire — are all present in food, human body humors, herbal products, and animal or inorganic compounds. These can be used to rectify the imbalance in the human body. In addition, the Siddha system treats the body as a temple and gives it a sacred status, stressing the need to take care diligently.

As in Ayurveda, Siddha also focuses on the normal equilibrium of three humors: Vatham, Pitham, and Kapham. The Siddha system recognises that 'food is medicine and medicine is food'.

Siddargal

Siddhars or Siddhargal were the premier scholars of this system in ancient India. Eighteen Siddhars were considered as the pillars of Siddha medicine. They wrote down their knowledge in many poems on dried palm leaves; these writings have been transcribed through many centuries.

Types of specialties

The Siddha system has many subspecialties. Kayakarpam is a combination of medicine and lifestyle. Varman therapy looks at the vital pressure points in the body that can be related to the illness. Vaasi (pranayama) looks at breathing strategies.

Medications in the Siddha system

Treatments in the Siddha system can be traced back to three origins: thavaram (plants), thadhu (inorganic substances) and jangamam (animals). Thadhu can be either uppu (salt types, water soluble), loham (water insoluble and melts on fire), pashanam (water insoluble, emits vapour on fire), uparasam (such as pashanam with different properties), rasam (soft) and gandhagam (metals or minerals, insoluble).

Evidence for Siddha medicine

Unfortunately, scientific evidence is lacking for many Siddha treatments. Case reports and low-quality evidence are available, but there is a lack of randomised controlled trials and systematic reviews. The Government of India has set up a Ministry of Ayush (Ayurveda, Yoga and naturopathy, Unani, Siddha, and Homeopathy) intending to produce proper evidence-based medicine from these traditional systems. Evidence has shown that the Siddha system concentrates on holistic aspects including lifestyle, dietary and environmental factors in developing various psychosomatic disorders.

Key Points

- The Siddha system of ancient traditional medicine originated from Tamil Nadu in South India.
- The Siddha refers to five basic elements: earth, sky, water, fire and sky; it recognises the need for equilibrium between Vatham, Pitham, and Kapham.
- Medications can be derived from plants, inorganic substances or animals.
- Scientific evidence is lacking for Siddha medicine due to a lack of high-quality trials.

References

1. National health portal India. Siddha medicine and treatment. Available from: http://www.nhp.gov.in/siddha_mty.

2. Wilson E, Rajamanickam GV, Vyas N, *et al.* Herbs used in Siddha medicine for arthritis – a review. *Indian J Trad Knowl* 2007; 6(4): 678-86.

3. Sood M, Singh SK, Chadda RK. Relevance of traditional Indian medical concepts in psychosomatic medicine. *Ann Natl Acad Med Sci (India)* 2017; 53(3): 148-55.

Fibromyalgia

Chapter 41

Homoeopathy

Introduction

Homoeopathy uses highly diluted substances that can heal the body. It is based on the theory of 'like cures like'; homoeopaths believe that a substance that causes disease in healthy people can cure similar symptoms in sick patients and administer these substances in diluted proportions. Claims for homoeopathy state that it works by stimulating the body's self-healing mechanisms. Homoeopathic substances can be of plant origin, but they differ from herbal remedies because they are given at extremely low concentrations.

A study quoted that more than 2% of the United States population use homoeopathy; musculoskeletal complaints are one of the main reasons for its use. However, only 19% of these users contacted a provider, while the rest relied on over-the-counter products. The most studied chronic pain condition in modern homoeopathic literature is fibromyalgia, but these studies still had significant flaws.

A 2010 House of Commons Science and Technology Committee report concluded that homoeopathic treatments are not better than giving placebos. The report concluded that doctors should not refer patients to homoeopaths for treatment.

Remedies

Homoeopathy states that each medicine should be individualised to each patient; the common homoeopathic remedies used in fibromyalgia include:

- *Arnica*: reduces bruising and swelling.
- *Bryonia* (vigorous vine, also called false mandrake): proposed to have anti-inflammatory actions.
- *Rhus toxicodendron* (poison ivy): proposed to relieve pain and stiffness.
- *Ruta grav*: less effective on stiffness.
- *Rhododendron*: less effective on pain related to stormy weather.
- Causticum: relieves pain, weakness, and stiffness, better in rainy weather.
- *Kalmia latifolia*: helps neuropathic shooting pain.
- *Cimicifuga*: for neck and upper back pain.

Evidence for homoeopathy

Unfortunately, there have been no high-quality randomised controlled trials for fibromyalgia; therefore it is impossible to recommend homoeopathy; at this time, only case reports are published in the literature.

A systematic review of homoeopathy in fibromyalgia found only four randomised trials, but all these reviews had severe flaws. Even though all studies favoured homoeopathy, the authors of the reviews looked at the flaws and quoted that the effectiveness of homoeopathy in fibromyalgia remains unproven.

Another review of homoeopathy in fibromyalgia looked at four randomised trials, one non-randomised trial, ten case reports and three observational studies; the case reports and observational studies did not have validated outcome measures. Meta-analyses revealed the benefits of homoeopathy regarding tender point count, pain intensity, and fatigue compared with placebo. However, the authors considered with caution that these results were preliminary.

The European League Against Rheumatism (EULAR) considered the systematic reviews in detail but noted the limitations of having only a small number of trials and the inherent flaws. Therefore, despite some benefits, due to the serious flaws, EULAR recommended strongly against the use of homoeopathy in fibromyalgia syndrome.

A German review in cooperation with eight medical, two psychological and two patient support groups looked at all the evidence. They concluded that homoeopathy could be recommended within a multicomponent therapy setting for a limited period.

A double-blinded controlled study of *Rhus toxicodendron 6c* found it beneficial in patients with fibromyalgia compared with a placebo, with high significance regarding the number of tender points.

Another randomised study of individualised homoeopathy treatment in fibromyalgia using a dilution factor of LM (1/50,000) daily showed improvements in tender point count, pain, quality of life, and global health compared with the administration of a placebo.

The need for more evidence

In summary, some homoeopathic studies have shown positive effects in patients with fibromyalgia, but these studies have serious flaws. As a result, the House of Commons Committee and EULAR have recommended against its use.

Key Points

- Homoeopathy uses highly diluted substances to cure ailments.
- Surveys show that many people use over-the-counter homoeopathic preparations rather than receiving treatment from a trained provider.
- Literature reports mainly describe the use of *Arnica, Bryonia* and *Rhus toxicodendron.*
- The evidence is limited as the studies on homoeopathy have significant flaws.
- EULAR recommends against the use of homoeopathy in fibromyalgia.

References

1.   National Health Service. Homeopathy. Available from: https://www.nhs.uk/conditions/homeopathy/.

2.   Dossett ML, Yeh GY. Homeopathy use in the United States and implications for public health: a review. *Homeopathy* 2018; 107(1): 3-9.

3.   House of Commons. Science and Technology Committee – Fourth Report. Evidence Check 2: Homeopathy. 2010. Available from: https://publications.parliament.uk/pa/cm200910/cmselect/cmsctech/45/4502.htm.

4.   Jones A. Fibromyalgia (FMS) can respond extremely well to homeopathy. Available from: https://homeopathy-uk.org/conditions-directory/fibromyalgia/.

5.   Perry R, Terry R, Ernst E. A systematic review of homeopathy for the treatment of fibromyalgia. *Clin Rheumatol* 2010; 29(5): 457-64.

6.   Boehm K, Raak C, Cramer H, *et al.* Homeopathy in the treatment of fibromyalgia – a comprehensive literature-review and meta-analysis. *Complement Ther Med* 2014; 22(4): 731-42.

7.   Macfarlane GJ, Kronisch C, Dean LE, *et al.* EULAR revised recommendations for the management of fibromyalgia. *Ann Rheum Dis* 2017; 76(2): 318-28.

8.   Langhorst J, Häuser W, Irnich D, *et al.* Alternative and complementary therapies in fibromyalgia syndrome. *Schmerz* 2008; 22(3): 324-33.

9.   Fisher P, Greenwood A, Huskisson EC, *et al.* Effect of homeopathic treatment on fibrositis (primary fibromyalgia). *BMJ* 1989; 299(6695): 365-6.

10. Bell IR, Lewis DA, Brooks AJ, *et al.* Improved clinical status in fibromyalgia patients treated with individualized homeopathic remedies versus placebo. *Rheumatology (Oxford)* 2004; 43(5): 577-82.

Section 7

Medications

Fibromyalgia

Chapter 42

Simple analgesics

Introduction

Patients commonly use painkillers for managing pain in fibromyalgia syndrome. This chapter deals with simple painkillers, including paracetamol and non-steroidal anti-inflammatory drugs (NSAIDs).

There is limited evidence on using simple analgesics in fibromyalgia, but most patients use over-the-counter medications for managing pain and flare-ups. A survey of 2596 patients with fibromyalgia conducted by the National Fibromyalgia Association in the USA showed that 67% of patients use over-the-counter medications and gave a median effectiveness score of 3.8 out of 10, proving that these patients continued to take these medications despite their low effectiveness. In addition, the survey showed that 94% of respondents used acetaminophen at some point and 37% continued to use it. In total, 87% had used ibuprofen in the past and 41% continued to use it; 66% had used naproxen before and 20% continued to use it; 48% had used celecoxib and 13% continued to use it.

Another survey of 800 patients and 1600 physicians from eight different countries found that 70% of these patients used pain medications prescribed by the physician and 36% used over-the-counter analgesics.

Paracetamol

Paracetamol (acetaminophen) is a simple analgesic and antipyretic drug available over the counter. Also known as N-acetyl-p-aminophenol, it is derived from phenol and has a core benzene ring structure. The maximum oral dose for adults is 1g taken every 4–6 hours (maximum dose of 4g in 24 hours). When taken orally, the onset of its analgesic effects is within 40 minutes, peaking after 1 hour. It has a good safety profile and effectiveness.

Pharmacology of paracetamol

Paracetamol inhibits prostaglandin E synthesis via the cyclo-oxygenase (COX) pathway and can also affect the nociceptive pathway. Several central and peripheral mechanisms of action have been suggested. It has an oral bioavailability of 70–90%, whereas rectal bioavailability is variable at approximately 40%. Paracetamol is metabolised in the liver primarily by glucuronidation. Cytochrome P450 enzymes oxidise a small fraction to form N-acetyl-p-benzoquinone imine (NAPQI), a toxic metabolite in paracetamol overdose, causing liver damage due to glutathione deficiency.

Paracetamol is used commonly for musculoskeletal pain relief, especially in the flare-up of fibromyalgia pain and during physiotherapy in rehabilitation.

Evidence for paracetamol

Unfortunately, there have been no high-quality studies or evidence for using paracetamol in fibromyalgia. Many existing studies have flaws and paracetamol is usually combined with other medications such as tramadol. The National Health Service (NHS) website still recommends paracetamol, mentioning that it can sometimes help relieve the pain associated with fibromyalgia. But the National Institute for Health and Clinical Excellence (NICE) guidelines in 2021 do not recommend paracetamol and NSAIDs for chronic primary pain.

A Cochrane review of combination pharmacotherapy concluded that there is no evidence to support or refute the use of combination pharmacotherapy for fibromyalgia.

A Spanish interdisciplinary consensus document looked at various treatments for fibromyalgia; it mentions that paracetamol and NSAIDs are the drugs most prescribed for fibromyalgia. The consensus notes that, in randomised trials, these medications have not been demonstrated to be superior to placebo. Therefore, the consensus group does not recommend these medications in patients with fibromyalgia, except if patients had any other associated disease in which these can be effective such as arthritis or soft tissue pain.

Non-steroidal anti-inflammatory drugs

NSAIDs are used in a variety of painful conditions and musculoskeletal pain.

They are classified as follows:

- Non-selective NSAIDs, including:
  - salicylates (aspirin);
  - acetic acid derivatives (diclofenac, ketorolac, indomethacin);
  - fenamates (mefenamic acid);
  - oxicam derivatives (meloxicam, piroxicam);
  - propionic acid derivatives (ibuprofen, naproxen).
- Selective COX-2 inhibitors, including pyrazoles (celecoxib, parecoxib, etoricoxib), have fewer gastrointestinal side effects. Some COX-2 inhibitors (rofecoxib and valdecoxib) have been withdrawn due to their cardiovascular side effects.

Topical NSAIDs are commonly used and available over the counter (e.g. ibuprofen gel, diclofenac gel) (please refer to Chapter 45 for more detail on topical agents).

NSAIDs act as COX inhibitors, reducing prostaglandin production; prostaglandins cause fever, pain and inflammatory responses (■ Figure

42.1). COX-1 is expressed constitutively, mediating prostaglandin production, and is involved in gastric mucosal protection, maintenance of renal blood flow and the synthesis of thromboxane (involved in platelet aggregation and vasoconstriction). Therefore, the main side effects of NSAIDs include gastric ulceration, renal damage and bleeding due to their inhibitory effects on COX.

COX-2 is an inducible form of the enzyme responsible for prostaglandin E2 (PGE2) production, which causes inflammatory responses and pain. However, COX-2-selective NSAIDs have fewer side effects.

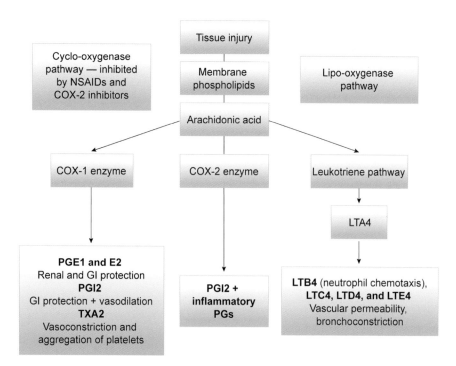

Figure 42.1. Mechanism of action of NSAIDs. COX-1 = cyclo-oxygenase-1; COX-2 = cyclo-oxygenase-2; LT = leukotriene; NSAID = non-steroidal anti-inflammatory drug; PG = prostaglandin; PGE1 = prostaglandin E1; PGE2 = prostaglandin E2; PGI2 = prostaglandin I2; TXA2 = thromboxane A2.

In addition to the side effects mentioned above, NSAIDs can precipitate bronchoconstriction in patients with asthma by stimulating the leukotriene pathway.

Ibuprofen should be taken at a maximum dose of 200–400mg orally three or four times daily on a full stomach, along with gastric protection, given its risk profile.

Evidence for NSAIDs

The European League Against Rheumatism (EULAR) identified only two small trials with no evidence of improvement in patients with fibromyalgia compared with placebo. The Committee cited weak evidence when advising against using NSAIDs in fibromyalgia. It is the one intervention in which the full committee (100%) agreed against the use of NSAIDs.

A Cochrane review of oral NSAIDs for fibromyalgia looked at six randomised, double-blinded trials with durations of treatment between 3 and 8 weeks; analyses consistently showed no significant difference between NSAIDs and placebo in fibromyalgia. Another Cochrane review found that pain reduction by half or better was experienced by 1 in 10 patients given NSAIDs and by 2 in 10 with placebo. Pain reduction by a third or better was experienced by 2 in 10 in both the NSAID and placebo groups. Side effects were experienced by 3 in 10 patients given NSAIDs and 2 in 10 patients given a placebo. A Cochrane review commented that the evidence was of very low quality.

Avoiding the use of simple analgesics as a routine in fibromyalgia

Paracetamol and NSAIDs cannot be recommended based on the available low-quality evidence in fibromyalgia syndrome. However, they can be used if the patient has co-existing arthritis or muscular pain. If an NSAID is administered, it should be used for a short duration at a small effective dose. As NSAIDs can cause significant gastric side effects, they should be reviewed and used sparingly.

Key Points

- Most patients with fibromyalgia have used or continue to use simple analgesics; a significant proportion of individuals use over-the-counter preparations.
- Low-quality evidence does not recommend paracetamol or NSAIDs in fibromyalgia.
- NSAIDs can cause significant side effects; caution should be taken to use a small effective dose for a short period, under regular review.

References

1. Bennett RM, Jones J, Turk DC, *et al*. An internet survey of 2,596 people with fibromyalgia. *BMC Musculoskelet Disord* 2007; 8: 27.

2. Choy E, Perrot S, Leon T, *et al*. A patient survey of the impact of fibromyalgia and the journey to diagnosis. *BMC Health Serv Res* 2010; 10: 102.

3. Crighton AJ, McCann CT, Todd EJ, Brown AJ. Safe use of paracetamol and high-dose NSAID analgesia in dentistry during the COVID-19 pandemic. *Br Dent J* 2020; 229(1): 15-8.

4. Vasu T. Simple medications. In: Vasu T. *Managing long COVID syndrome*. Shrewsbury, UK: tfm publishing Ltd; 2022: pp. 217-20.

5. Ingle PM. Pharmacology — non-steroidal anti-inflammatory drugs (NSAIDs). In: Vasu T, Balasubramanian S, Kodivalasa M, Ingle PM, Eds. *Chronic pain management*. Shrewsbury, UK: tfm publishing Ltd; 2021: pp. 223-33.

6. National Health Service. Treatment – fibromyalgia. Available from: https://www.nhs.uk/conditions/fibromyalgia/treatment/#:~:text=Simple%20painkillers%20that%20are%20available,the%20medication%20before%20using%20them.

7. National Institute for Health and Care Excellence; 2021. Chronic pain (primary and secondary) in over 16s: assessment of all chronic pain and management of chronic primary pain. NICE guideline, NG193. Available from: https://www.nice.org.uk/guidance/ng193/chapter/Recommendations#managing-chronic-primary-pain.

8. Thorpe J, Shum B, Moore RA, *et al*. Combination pharmacotherapy for the treatment of fibromyalgia in adults. *Cochrane Database Syst Rev* 2018; 2: CD010585.

9.   de Miquel CA, Campayo JG, Flórez MT, *et al.* Interdisciplinary consensus document for the treatment of fibromyalgia. *Actas Esp Psiquiatr* 2010; 38(2): 108-20.

10.   Macfarlane GJ, Kronisch C, Dean LE, *et al.* EULAR revised recommendations for the management of fibromyalgia. *Ann Rheum Dis* 2017; 76(2): 318-28.

11.   Derry S, Wiffen PJ, Häuser W, *et al.* Oral nonsteroidal anti-inflammatory drugs for fibromyalgia in adults. *Cochrane Database Syst Rev* 2017; 3: CD012332.

Fibromyalgia

Chapter 43

Neuropathic medications

Introduction

Neuropathic medications are trialled commonly in patients with fibromyalgia, but they only have limited efficacy. Patients need to be educated on the characteristics of these medications, need for follow-up and plans to review and be advised when to stop treatments if they do not help the condition. Many failures of pharmacological therapy are due to a lack of patient education and follow-up. Any medication that has not improved the quality of life or pain should be stopped after an adequate trial period rather than continuing treatment inappropriately.

An internet survey of 2596 patients undertaken by the National Fibromyalgia Association in the USA showed that 55% of respondents had used amitriptyline in the past, 42% found them to be helpful, and 22% continued to still use them. The same survey also showed that 36% of respondents continued to use gabapentin and 46% of the respondents found it to be helpful.

Tricyclic antidepressants

Tricyclic antidepressants, including amitriptyline and nortriptyline, are the first-line choice for the management of neuropathic pain, according to the National Institute for Health and Care Excellence (NICE) guidelines. Their mechanism of action is via inhibition of presynaptic reuptake of noradrenaline and serotonin. In neuropathic pain, the number needed to treat (NNT) is 3.6.

Tricyclic antidepressants are metabolised in the liver and excreted by the kidneys. They are contraindicated in arrhythmias, the manic phase of bipolar disorder, heart block and immediately following myocardial infarction. Side effects manifest as anticholinergic (dry mouth, constipation, blurred vision, urinary retention), antihistaminergic (drowsiness) and anti-alpha-adrenergic (low blood pressure, prolonged QT interval and atrioventricular block) responses.

The drugs are taken orally once daily at 10–75mg doses. Patients should initially be given a small dose, which is then slowly increased, as needed, depending on the side effects. Advice indicates that tricyclic antidepressants should be taken in the early evening to avoid drowsiness on waking in the morning. In addition, dry mouth can be persistent and patients should be advised regarding adequate hydration.

Evidence for amitriptyline in fibromyalgia

A systematic review of amitriptyline in patients with fibromyalgia looking at ten moderate-quality to high-quality randomised trials concluded that there was some evidence to support the short-term use of amitriptyline at 25mg/day. However, there was no evidence to support amitriptyline at higher doses or for periods of more than 8 weeks.

The European League Against Rheumatism (EULAR) looked at five reviews that included 13 studies and quoted weak evidence that supported amitriptyline administered at a low dose for fibromyalgia; there was a 100% agreement of the Committee for this support for amitriptyline in fibromyalgia.

Gabapentinoids

Gabapentinoids bind to the α2δ (alpha-2 delta) subunit of voltage-gated calcium channels, resulting in a reduction in presynaptic calcium influx, thereby reducing the release of excitatory neurotransmitters (such as glutamate, substance P and calcitonin gene-related peptide [CGRP]) from neuronal tissues.

Pregabalin is more potent than gabapentin. Pregabalin has a better pharmacokinetic profile, better bioavailability and a longer duration of action compared with gabapentin. In neuropathic pain, the number needed to treat (NNT) for gabapentinoids is 4.2–6.4.

Central nervous system side effects, pedal oedema, increased body weight and gastrointestinal side effects are common following gabapentinoid use.

Gabapentin is taken orally and started at 300mg once daily, then increased gradually to a usual dose of 600mg three times daily. Smaller doses can be trialled if side effects occur.

Pregabalin is taken orally and started at 25mg or 75mg once daily, depending on the patient's weight, and increased gradually, up to a maximum dose of 300mg twice daily. After a trial of 4–6 weeks, if gabapentinoids have not helped, patients should be gradually weaned off them. Starting at low doses that are increased slowly is the key to success in drug therapy for chronic pain.

In the UK, due to potential misuse, these drugs are classified as Class C controlled drugs, meaning they are available only by a prescription issued by a qualified healthcare professional.

Evidence for gabapentinoids in fibromyalgia

An updated Cochrane review published in 2017 concluded that the evidence was insufficient to give definite conclusions on the efficacy and safety of gabapentin, lacosamide and levetiracetam in fibromyalgia. The use of pregabalin demonstrated a small benefit over placebo in pain and sleep domains. Dizziness was frequently found following pregabalin administration and study dropout rates were higher. It was noted that pregabalin did not improve fatigue or reduce disability.

In 2017, another updated Cochrane review of gabapentin for chronic neuropathic pain concluded that the evidence in fibromyalgia was limited. In addition, it mentions that over half of those treated with gabapentin did not have worthwhile pain relief and also experienced adverse events. These events included dizziness (19%), somnolence (14%), peripheral oedema (7%) and gait disturbance (14%).

The EULAR supported pregabalin with weak evidence for patients with fibromyalgia; it recommended that gabapentin be used only for research.

Serotonin-noradrenaline reuptake inhibitors

Serotonin-noradrenaline reuptake inhibitors (SNRIs), such as duloxetine, are used for treating neuropathic pain and are recommended by NICE guidelines. They inhibit presynaptic serotonin and noradrenaline reuptake. In neuropathic pain conditions, the number needed to treat (NNT) is 6.4. Duloxetine treatment produced a 3–10 times selective inhibition of serotonin reuptake compared with norepinephrine reuptake.

SNRIs are usually taken orally; duloxetine can be started at a dose of 30–60mg once daily, which is then increased to a maximum dose of 120mg daily. Side effects include sleep problems, headache, dizziness, blurred vision and dry mouth.

Milnacipran is used less often in the UK. However, in 2009 it was approved by the United States Food and Drug Administration (US FDA) for use in the USA for fibromyalgia. Milnacipran has a greater norepinephrine reuptake ratio than duloxetine (reuptake of serotonin and norepinephrine in the ratio of 1:3 to 1:1).

Evidence for SNRIs in fibromyalgia

A Cochrane review (2014) on duloxetine concluded that there was low-quality evidence that SNRIs were effective in fibromyalgia at doses of 60–120mg per day. In addition, the review mentioned that the effect of this medication in fibromyalgia could be achieved through a greater improvement in mental symptoms than in somatic physical pain. The NNT for duloxetine in fibromyalgia was 8.

An updated Cochrane review (2018) looked at the use of SNRIs in fibromyalgia. Based on low-quality to very-low-quality evidence, the SNRIs duloxetine and milnacipran provided no benefit over placebo for pain relief of 50% or greater. However, if pain relief of 30% or more was calculated, there was a clinically relevant benefit and an improvement in the Patients' Global Impression of Change (PGIC) score. There was no improvement in health-related quality of life, sleep or reducing fatigue. The potential benefits of duloxetine and milnacipran in fibromyalgia were outweighed by their potential harm. In a minority of people with fibromyalgia, duloxetine and milnacipran might give substantial pain relief without adverse events.

The EULAR gave support with weak evidence for the use of duloxetine in fibromyalgia.

A Cochrane review (2015) looked at randomised studies of 8–24 weeks' duration. The review found that milnacipran at a dose of 100mg or 200mg was effective only in a minority of patients with fibromyalgia, giving 30% pain relief to approximately 40% of participants, compared with 30% with placebo. This gave an NNT of 6–10 for an additional beneficial outcome. It was associated with increased adverse events, especially with higher doses; the number needed to harm (NNH) was 23 with a 100mg dose, which worsened to nine with a 200mg dose. The NNH was 5.7 for nausea, 13 for constipation and 29 for headache on average, as described in the review.

Selective serotonin reuptake inhibitors (SSRIs)

SSRI drugs have been studied previously but not found to be beneficial for treating neuropathic pain. These include drugs such as citalopram, fluoxetine, paroxetine and sertraline. Therefore, based on the weak evidence, the EULAR advised against using SSRIs in fibromyalgia.

NICE guidelines for neuropathic pain

NICE guidance on neuropathic pain recommends using amitriptyline, gabapentin, pregabalin or duloxetine. If the initial treatment with one drug is ineffective, another drug from the list should be used.

For acute rescue therapy, the guidance recommends the use of tramadol and also capsaicin cream for localised neuropathic pain.

Other evidence

German guidelines strongly recommend using amitriptyline (dose of 25–50mg/day) with a grade A recommendation (grade 1a evidence, level 1 intervention). However, based on a grade B recommendation (grade 1a evidence), they supported short-term use of pregabalin (150–300mg/day), duloxetine (60–120mg/day) and milnacipran (100–200mg/day) with a majority opinion (level 3 interventions) rather than strong consensus.

A Cochrane review of carbamazepine in patients with fibromyalgia found no trials longer than 4 weeks' duration or of good reporting quality. Carbamazepine is probably effective in some patients, but caution was needed when interpreting the low-quality evidence. A Cochrane review of lacosamide could not find adequate data on fibromyalgia to analyse. It was likely that lacosamide had no useful benefit in neuropathic pain and any positive interpretation should be made with caution. A Cochrane review of lamotrigine in fibromyalgia did not show any convincing evidence that it was effective. It concluded that lamotrigine did not have a significant role based on the available evidence for fibromyalgia; there was concern about an adverse effect profile.

Evidence comparing drugs

A systematic review compared amitriptyline, duloxetine and milnacipran in patients with fibromyalgia; it concluded that amitriptyline could not be recommended as the gold standard for fibromyalgia treatment with antidepressants because of the methodological limitations of the studies. However, it found that the quality of studies on duloxetine and milnacipran was high. The effects of all three medications were superior to those of placebo in most domains.

Placebo response with medications

A systematic review looked at pharmacological therapy in fibromyalgia from 72 studies of 9827 patients; they calculated the pooled weighted mean difference between pain baseline and end of treatment scores in the active drug group and the placebo group using a random effects model. The placebo response accounted for 45% of the response of the fibromyalgia group. In addition, the placebo response was associated with the year of study initiation, pain baseline and effect size in the active group; the placebo response was not associated with age, sex and race.

Core principle of pain pharmacotherapy

An analysis published in the *British Medical Journal* clarified a study on pregabalin in fibromyalgia; pain relief was not normally distributed but usually bimodal, being either very good (above 50%) or poor (below 15%). Therefore, averaging pain relief is not helpful when analysing the effect of medication.

The author of this article stated that it was important that clinicians who treated patients with fibromyalgia should be ready to expect and recognise analgesic failure and react to it, rather than blindly accepting failure. The article concluded with a few key points that are important for every clinician facing a patient with fibromyalgia:

- A single drug only helps a minority of patients with fibromyalgia.
- Successful pain relief also helps to improve sleep, function, mood, fatigue, quality of life and the ability to work.
- The failure of one drug does not necessarily mean failure with others, even within a class.
- We do not know the best order in which to prescribe drugs.
- Success or failure is evidenced within 2–4 weeks and, if achieved, tends to be long lasting. The clinician needs to review treatment at that time and decide if the patient needs to continue with the medication or not, after an active dialogue with the patient and assessment of the various modalities of the outcome.

Review of neuropathic medications in fibromyalgia

Given that the NNT for most neuropathic medications, in general, is between 4 and 6, after a few weeks the clinician needs to review whether the medication has been effective. All medications work only in some and not all. This should be clearly explained to the patients before treatment starts and reviewed at appropriate intervals. If it has not helped, either the dose needs to be changed or additive medications advised, or the medication should be stopped. This plan should be clearly explained before treatment starts, to let the patient participate in this comprehensive plan. In summary, after a trial of 4–6 weeks of drug treatment, it is important to review the patient to assess the efficacy and side effects of the treatment.

Key Points

- The NNT for tricyclic antidepressants in neuropathic pain is 3.6.
- The evidence supports the use of low-dose amitriptyline in fibromyalgia, but the long-term outcome is unclear.
- Gabapentinoids have an NNT of 4–6; the evidence is limited, but the EULAR supports pregabalin with weak evidence.
- Regarding SNRIs, duloxetine has an NNT of 6–8; low-quality evidence supports its use in fibromyalgia.
- A single drug only helps a minority of patients with fibromyalgia syndrome; use needs to be reviewed at 2–4 weeks' duration.
- Failure of one drug does not mean failure with another drug, even within the same class.

References

1. Bennett RM, Jones J, Turk DC, *et al.* An internet survey of 2,596 people with fibromyalgia. *BMC Musculoskelet Disord* 2007; 8: 27.

2. National Institute for Health and Care Excellence; 2013. Neuropathic pain in adults: pharmacological management in nonspecialist settings. Clinical guideline CG173. Available from: https://www.nice.org.uk/guidance/cg173.

3. Vasu T. Neuropathic pain medications. In: Vasu T. *Managing long COVID syndrome*. Shrewsbury, UK: tfm publishing Ltd; 2022: pp. 221-4.

4. Murally H, Ingle PM. Pharmacology — other anti-neuropathic agents. In: Vasu T, Balasubramanian S, Kodivalasa M, Ingle PM, Eds. *Chronic pain management*. Shrewsbury, UK: tfm publishing Ltd; 2021: pp. 255-62.

5. Ingle PM. Pharmacology — gabapentinoids. In: Vasu T, Balasubramanian S, Kodivalasa M, Ingle PM, Eds. *Chronic pain management*. Shrewsbury, UK: tfm publishing Ltd; 2021: pp. 249-54.

6. Nishishinya B, Urrútia G, Walitt B, *et al.* Amitriptyline in the treatment of fibromyalgia: a systematic review of its efficacy. *Rheumatology (Oxford)* 2008; 47(12): 1741-6.

7. Macfarlane GJ, Kronisch C, Dean LE, *et al.* EULAR revised recommendations for the management of fibromyalgia. *Ann Rheum Dis* 2017; 76(2): 318-28.

8. Üçeyler N, Sommer C, Walitt B, Häuser W. Anticonvulsants for fibromyalgia. *Cochrane Database Syst Rev* 2013; 2017(10): CD010782.

9. Wiffen PJ, Derry S, Bell RF, *et al.* Gabapentin for chronic neuropathic pain in adults. *Cochrane Database Syst Rev* 2017; 6(6): CD007938.

10. Lunn MPT, Hughes RAC, Wiffen PJ. Duloxetine for treating painful neuropathy, chronic pain or fibromyalgia. *Cochrane Database Syst Rev* 2014; 1(1): CD007115.

11. Welsch P, Üçeyler N, Klose P, *et al.* Serotonin and noradrenaline reuptake inhibitors (SNRIs) for fibromyalgia. *Cochrane Database Syst Rev* 2018; 2(2): CD010292.

12. Cording M, Derry S, Phillips T, *et al.* Milnacipran for pain in fibromyalgia in adults. *Cochrane Database Syst Rev* 2015; 2015(10): CD008244.

13. Häuser W, Eich W, Herrmann M, *et al.* Fibromyalgia syndrome: classification, diagnosis, and treatment. *Dtsch Arztebl Int* 2009; 106(23): 383-91.

14. Wiffen PJ, Derry S, Moore RA, Kalso EA. Carbamazepine for chronic neuropathic pain and fibromyalgia in adults. *Cochrane Database Syst Rev* 2014; (4): CD005451.

15. Hearn L, Derry S, Moore RA. Lacosamide for neuropathic pain and fibromyalgia in adults. *Cochrane Database Syst Rev* 2012; (2): CD009318.

16. Wiffen PJ, Derry S, Moore RA. Lamotrigine for chronic neuropathic pain and fibromyalgia in adults. *Cochrane Database Syst Rev* 2013; (12): CD006044.

17. Häuser W, Petzke F, Üçeyler N, Sommer C. Comparative efficacy and acceptability of amitriptyline, duloxetine and milnacipran in fibromyalgia syndrome: a systematic review with meta-analysis. *Rheumatology (Oxford)* 2011; 50(3): 532-43.

18.   Häuser W, Bartram-Wunn E, Bartram C, *et al.* Systematic review: placebo response in drug trials of fibromyalgia syndrome and painful peripheral diabetic neuropathy – magnitude and patient-related predictors. *Pain* 2011; 152(8): 1709-17.

19.   Moore A, Derry S, Eccleston C, Kalso E. Expect analgesic failure; pursue analgesic success. *BMJ* 2013; 346: f2690.

Chapter 44

Opioids

Introduction

In managing fibromyalgia syndrome, opioids can become a problem rather than be a solution. Although there is a range of very good opioid analgesics for treating acute pain, evidence for their long-term use in fibromyalgia is limited. However, a patient survey by the Fibromyalgia Association in the USA found that patients considered them the most helpful drugs among prescribed medications (75% for hydrocodone and 67% for oxycodone).

The Faculty of Pain Medicine's guidelines *Opioids Aware* explains that initiating, tapering or stopping opioid treatment should be made in agreement with the patient, their general practitioner/family doctor and all members of the healthcare team involved in the patient's management.

Opioid pharmacology

Opioid receptors are classified into four major types: mu (μ) opioid (MOP), kappa (κ) opioid (KOP), delta (δ) opioid (DOP) and nociceptin/orphanin FQ (N/OFQ). Opioid receptors are linked to inhibitory G-proteins and, on activation, close voltage-gated calcium channels, causing hyperpolarisation by potassium efflux and inhibiting adenylyl cyclase. This leads to decreased cyclic adenosine monophosphate (cAMP) and a reduced release of neurotransmitters. Opioid medications inhibit the ascending excitatory pathway and activate the descending inhibitory pathway.

Common opioids

Morphine
Morphine has an oral bioavailability of 30% due to high first-pass metabolism. Given as an intravenous bolus, it has peak action after 10 minutes. It is metabolised by glucuronidation in the liver and gut; it is excreted via the kidneys and bile. Morphine-6-glucuronide can accumulate and lead to liver failure. The side effects of morphine include respiratory depression, reduced response to carbon dioxide, suppression of cough response, hypotension, bradycardia, histamine release, sphincter of Oddi contraction and reduced levels of endocrine hormones (such as adrenocorticotrophic hormone), prolactin and gonadotrophic hormones.

Codeine
Codeine, or 3-methylmorphine, is a prodrug and a weak opioid. It is metabolised by glucuronidation. It undergoes N-demethylation to norcodeine. Approximately 10% undergoes O-demethylation to morphine, with good analgesic effects, under the influence of the cytochrome P450 enzyme (CYP2D6). Unfortunately, CYP2D6 is absent in approximately 10% of the white population, in whom, therefore, codeine does not provide effective analgesia.

Oxycodone
Oxycodone is a MOP receptor agonist and a semi-synthetic derivative of thebaine. It has nearly twice the oral bioavailability of morphine. It is metabolised by N- and O-demethylation to noroxycodone and normorphine, respectively.

Tramadol
Tramadol is a racemic mixture of two stereoisomers; it is a weak opioid with mild SNRI activity. It works as a MOP receptor agonist, reducing neuronal reuptake of serotonin. It is helpful in treating neuropathic pain. The National Institute for Health and Care Excellence (NICE) guidelines for treating neuropathic pain recommend adding tramadol to other neuropathic

pain medications. Tramadol is metabolised in the liver; it can interact with tricyclic antidepressants and SSRIs causing serotonergic syndrome.

Fentanyl
Fentanyl is a selective MOP receptor agonist with a rapid onset of action. It is 100 times more potent than morphine. Transdermal fentanyl is used in treating chronic pain but produces significant side effects at high doses, as is the case with any opioid. Fentanyl has high solubility and is rapidly redistributed. Its side effects include chest wall rigidity and bronchospasm.

Buprenorphine
Buprenorphine is a semi-synthetic partial MOP agonist and a KOP antagonist. It also has agonist effects on the N/OFQ receptor. It is more potent than morphine and has a longer duration of action due to its high receptor affinity. Therefore it is commonly used as a transdermal preparation.

Common side effects

Common side effects of opioids include respiratory depression, constipation, drowsiness, confusion, nausea and tolerance. Of particular concern is the physical dependence on opioids, an important side effect of this drug class.

Reduced efficacy in fibromyalgia

Opioids have not shown benefits in many studies on fibromyalgia. Looking at μ-opioid receptor (MOR) positron emission tomography, a study demonstrated that there was altered endogenous opioid activity in patients with fibromyalgia; this could explain the reduced efficacy of exogenous opioids in fibromyalgia. Patients with fibromyalgia had reduced MOR binding potential within many areas involved in pain modulation, including the nucleus accumbens, the amygdala and the dorsal cingulate.

Warnings of long-term use of high-dose opioids

The evidence for opioid use in the long term, especially at high doses, is limited. However, studies have reported significant harm, which has led to the creation of various guidelines to educate providers on the harms of opioid use. The Faculty of Pain Medicine of the Royal College of Anaesthetists has published the *Opioids Aware* guidelines to educate all healthcare professionals. The risk of harm from opioid use increases substantially at doses of more than 120mg morphine equivalent per day. Help from a multidisciplinary team should be sought for at-risk patients.

Harm from long-term opioid use

Long-term opioid use at high doses causes endocrine and immunological problems and reduces bone density. Furthermore, long-term, high-dose opioid use can also lead to opioid-induced allodynia in which opioids themselves can cause pain; this is due to changes in neuroplasticity at the opioid receptor level.

Sleep problems in fibromyalgia

Opioids can disrupt sleep patterns and architecture; a polysomnography study of 193 fibromyalgia and insomnia patients showed that opioids increased lighter sleep (stage 2) and reduced slow-wave sleep. This sleep disruption was exacerbated at higher opioid doses in older adults and patients with low pain.

Opioids attenuate other beneficial interventions

A randomised controlled trial analysed the benefits of motivational interviewing in patients with fibromyalgia and divided these into two groups of opioid users and non-users. There was no benefit of motivational interviewing in opioid users. However, in non-opioid-using patients with fibromyalgia, there was a significant improvement in physical function, pain severity and global fibromyalgia severity with motivational interviewing, and the benefits were sustained for 6 months after completion of the therapy.

Evidence for opioids in fibromyalgia

A systematic review looking at the use of opioids in patients with fibromyalgia concluded that there was no evidence that opioids were effective in fibromyalgia and expressed the need for caution. In addition, it found that observational studies in fibromyalgia showed that opioid-receiving patients have poorer outcomes than non-opioid groups.

The European League Against Rheumatism (EULAR) looked at the efficacy of tramadol in fibromyalgia and considered two reviews; with weak evidence, it supports the role of tramadol in fibromyalgia. However, the EULAR commented that it did not identify any reviews on opioids in fibromyalgia. However, the EULAR Committee made a 'strong against' evaluation for the use of strong opioids in fibromyalgia (100% agreement), based on the lack of evidence and the high risk of side effects/addiction reported in individual trials.

A prospective cohort study with a 2-year longitudinal follow-up of patients with fibromyalgia in a multidisciplinary centre found that opioids were associated with negative health-related measures. The outcomes were poorer regarding symptoms, functional status and occupational status than non-users. Patients with fibromyalgia who were treated with opioids were more symptomatic, more likely to be unemployed and more likely to be receiving disability benefits.

An observational study in a tertiary care multidisciplinary fibromyalgia clinic showed that 32% of referred patients were using opioids, with more than two-thirds using strong opioids. In this study, opioid use was associated with lower education, unemployment, disability payments, unstable psychiatric disorders, a history of substance abuse and previous suicide attempts. In addition, they concluded that opioid use resulted in negative health and psychosocial status in patients with fibromyalgia.

In another 12-month observational study of 1700 patients with fibromyalgia, opioid users showed less improvement in outcome measures than the non-opioid group. These findings did not support the use of opioids in fibromyalgia. However, tramadol treatment produced better outcomes than other opioids.

A tertiary pain rehabilitation centre looked at the retrospective data of 159 patients with fibromyalgia who had completed a 3-week outpatient opioid weaning programme. Patients taking opioids had a morphine equivalent mean dose of 99mg/day. This programme involved tapering opioids over a mean of 10 days if the daily morphine equivalent dose was less than 100mg/day. The programme tapered use over a mean of 28 days if the patients were on doses of more than 200mg/day. There were no differences in withdrawal symptoms based on the opioid dose; the duration of opioid use did not affect the time to complete the opioid taper or withdrawal symptoms. After patients were weaned off opioids, they showed significant improvement in pain scores, depression catastrophising, health perception, interference with life and perceived life control.

Role of opioid antagonists

Case reports have shown a benefit when administering a low dose of the opioid antagonist, naltrexone, in patients with fibromyalgia. However, based on the proposed endocrine theory in fibromyalgia aetiology, authors of a case report claimed that exogenous opioids would suppress the endorphin system and worsen fibromyalgia symptoms.

Another pilot cross-over study of low-dose naltrexone showed a greater than 30% reduction in symptoms in patients with fibromyalgia compared with individuals given a placebo. Naltrexone is proposed to inhibit microglia activity and reverse central and peripheral inflammation. The beneficial response was maintained for approximately 2 weeks after treatment was stopped.

Key Points

- Opioids can become a problem rather than a solution in chronic pain conditions such as fibromyalgia syndrome.
- The *Opioids Aware* guidelines from the Faulty of Pain Medicine, UK, have helped to direct opioid management in these patients.
- Opioids can disrupt the sleep pattern in patients with fibromyalgia.
- Multidisciplinary help should be sought if the daily dose exceeds 120mg/day of morphine equivalent.
- The evidence does not support the use of opioids in fibromyalgia; studies have shown poorer outcomes.
- The EULAR Committee strongly recommends against the use of opioids in patients with fibromyalgia.

References

1. Bennett RM, Jones J, Turk DC, *et al.* An internet survey of 2596 people with fibromyalgia. *BMC Musculoskelet Disord* 2007; 8: 27.

2. Rajan RS, Ingle PM. Pharmacology — opioids. In: Vasu T, Balasubramanian S, Kodivalasa M, Ingle PM, Eds. *Chronic pain management.* Shrewsbury, UK: tfm publishing Ltd; 2021: pp. 235-44.

3. Vasu T. Harmful effects of opioids. In: Vasu T. *Managing long COVID syndrome.* Shrewsbury, UK: tfm publishing Ltd; 2022: pp. 225-9.

4. Vasu T. Problems of opioid use in chronic pain. In: Vasu T, Balasubramanian S, Kodivalasa M, Ingle PM, Eds. *Chronic pain management.* Shrewsbury, UK: tfm publishing Ltd; 2021: pp. 245-8.

5. National Institute for Health and Care Excellence; 2013. Neuropathic pain in adults: pharmacological management in nonspecialist settings. Clinical guideline CG173. Available from: https://www.nice.org.uk/guidance/cg173.

6. Faculty of Pain Medicine. Opioids aware. Available from: https://www.fpm.ac.uk/opioids-aware.

7. Harris RE, Clauw DJ, Scott DJ, *et al.* Decreased central μ-opioid receptor availability in fibromyalgia. *J Neurosci* 2007; 27(37): 10000-6.

8. Curtis AF, Miller MB, Rathinakumar H, *et al.* Opioid use, pain intensity, age, and sleep architecture in patients with fibromyalgia and insomnia. *Pain* 2019; 160(9): 2086-92.

9. Kim S, Slaven JE, Ang DC. Sustained benefits of exercise-based motivational interviewing, but only among nonusers of opioids in patients with fibromyalgia. *J Rheumatol* 2017; 44(4): 505-11.

10. Goldenberg DL, Clauw DJ, Palmer RE, Clair AG. Opioid use in fibromyalgia: a cautionary tale. *Mayo Clin Proc* 2016; 91(5): 640-8.

11. Macfarlane GJ, Kronisch C, Dean LE, *et al*. EULAR revised recommendations for the management of fibromyalgia. *Ann Rheum Dis* 2017; 76(2): 318-28.

12. Fitzcharles M, Faregh N, Ste-Marie PA, Shir Y. Opioid use in fibromyalgia is associated with negative health related measures in a prospective cohort study. *Pain Res Treat* 2013; 2013: ID898493.

13. Fitzcharles MA, Ste-Marie PA, Gamsa A, *et al*. Opioid use, misuse, and abuse in patients labeled as fibromyalgia. *Am J Med* 2011; 124(10): 955-60.

14. Peng X, Robinson RL, Mease P, *et al*. Long-term evaluation of opioid treatment in fibromyalgia. *Clin J Pain* 2015; 31(1): 7-13.

15. Cunningham JL, Evans MM, King SM, *et al*. Opioid tapering in fibromyalgia patients: experience from an interdisciplinary pain rehabilitation program. *Pain Med* 2016; 17(9): 1676-85.

16. Ramanathan S, Panksepp J, Johnson B. Is fibromyalgia an endocrine/endorphin deficit disorder? Is low dose naltrexone a new treatment option? *Psychosomatics* 2012; 53(6): 591-4.

17. Younger J, Mackey S. Fibromyalgia symptoms are reduced by low-dose naltrexone: a pilot study. *Pain Med* 2009; 10(4): 663-72.

Chapter 45

Topical agents

Introduction

Fibromyalgia presents with widespread pain all over the body, but many patients have relied on topical medications to help their localised pain. Topical agents have a higher patient satisfaction rate and can reduce the systemic side effects of pharmacological products with clinically insignificant serum levels.

Topical heat or cold packs

A survey of patients with fibromyalgia showed that 74% of patients used hot packs or other heat modalities. This approach was claimed to be one of the highest effective interventions (effectiveness score of 6.3 on a 0–10 scale). However, cold therapy such as ice packs or pads was used only in 30% of patients with fibromyalgia and scored an effectiveness scale of 4.8.

Topical creams

Topical lidocaine cream
A 4% or 5% preparation of topical lidocaine cream is available over the counter for local anaesthetic action and can be applied three times a day.

Topical creams differ from transdermal patches because serum drug concentration is minimal; in transdermal patches, the drug concentration in blood is higher.

A Cochrane review of topical lidocaine looked at various formulations, including 5% cream, 5% gel, 8% spray and 5% transdermal medicated patches in neuropathic pain. The review did not find any evidence to support the use of topical lidocaine in neuropathic pain, although individual studies indicated that it was effective for pain relief.

Topical NSAID cream

Topical NSAIDs are commonly used in chronic musculoskeletal localised pain conditions rather than for widespread pain. The Scottish Intercollegiate Guidelines Network (SIGN) guidelines recommend NSAID cream for chronic pain from musculoskeletal conditions, particularly in patients who cannot tolerate oral NSAIDs.

Topical capsaicin cream

Capsaicin is trans-8-methyl-N-vanillyl-6-nonenamide and is a component of chilli pepper. It acts on the transient receptor potential vanilloid 1 (TRPV-1) receptor and can cause depletion of substance P from presynaptic terminals. In addition, it can reduce pain-related epidermal nerve fibres and results in neurodegeneration.

Topical capsaicin 0.025% and 0.075% have been used for localised neuropathic pain rather than widespread pain; 8% capsaicin patches also have a role in regional or localised neuropathic pain. The capsaicin 8% patch (Qutenza®) is 14cm x 20cm in dimension and contains 179mg capsaicin or 640µg/cm^2.

Topical plasters

Lidocaine 5% plaster

A 5% topical lidocaine plaster contains 700mg equivalent of a local anaesthetic applied over painful areas. It should only be applied for 12 hours and then removed for the next 12 hours. Patients should be informed repeatedly, to understand the necessity of this safety precaution. The manufacturer advises restricting application to a maximum of three plasters at a time. Many clinicians even advise cutting the plasters as needed to avoid side effects.

Lidocaine plasters work locally with a sodium channel blockade effect.

It is contraindicated if there is a history of allergy to lidocaine or other local anaesthetics. Plasters should not be applied over open wounds or broken skin. Caution should be taken if the patient has severe heart, kidney or liver disease.

Many healthcare regulators try to restrict the use of topical lidocaine plasters for regional neuropathic pain only rather than for widespread pain.

Topical opioid transdermal delivery systems

Buprenorphine (BuTrans® 5–20µg/hour or Butec® 35µg/hour) and fentanyl (12.5µg/hour or more) have been trialled in various chronic pain conditions but have significant opioid limitations and side effects. Opioids have a limited role in fibromyalgia syndrome; please refer to Chapter 44 for more detail.

Other topical agents

Topical rubefacients have been used in musculoskeletal conditions if other pharmacological therapies are ineffective. SIGN guidelines quote an NNT of 6.2 in musculoskeletal pain.

Topical menthol works on cold receptor areas of TRPM-8 receptors and can help in musculoskeletal pain.

Case reports have described the beneficial effects of topical amitriptyline and topical gabapentin, although it is not in common use.

Topical cannabidiol has been studied, but the evidence does not support its use in fibromyalgia; please refer to Chapter 47 for more detail.

Key Points

- There is no evidence for topical agents in fibromyalgia, but these continue to be used by patients for localised pain.

- Various topical agents work through different mechanisms, but these agents have limited efficacy in the widespread pain found in fibromyalgia syndrome.

References

1. Bennett RM, Jones J, Turk DC, *et al.* An internet survey of 2,596 people with fibromyalgia. *BMC Musculoskelet Disord* 2007; 8: 27.

2. Derry S, Wiffen PJ, Moore RA, Quinlan J. Topical lidocaine for neuropathic pain in adults. *Cochrane Database Syst Rev* 2014; 7(7): CD010958.

3. Health improvement Scotland. SIGN 136: management of chronic pain; Dec 2013. Available from: http://www.sign.ac.uk/assets/sign136.pdf.

4. Puttappa A, Ingle PM. Pharmacology – topical agents. In: Vasu T, Balasubramanian S, Kodivalasa M, Ingle PM, Eds. *Chronic pain management*. Shrewsbury, UK: tfm publishing Ltd; 2021: pp. 271-9.

Chapter 46

NMDA antagonists

Introduction

N-methyl-D-aspartate (NMDA) receptor antagonists are used in different types of chronic pain and have also been trialled in fibromyalgia syndrome. However, they have significant dissociative anaesthetic, hallucinogenic and euphoriant properties limiting their use.

Mechanism of action

Scientific evidence shows that NMDA receptors have increased activity in fibromyalgia; the modulation of these receptors by antagonists can help with pain and symptom management in fibromyalgia.

Increased sensitivity at the spinal cord neuron level in fibromyalgia is proposed to involve nociceptive input via C- and A-delta fibres. In addition, deeply placed polymodal neurons receive mechanoreceptor input; these are dependent on NMDA receptor activity.

Studies have shown elevated levels of glutamate (GluN) in the brain of patients with fibromyalgia; this was shown to correlate with pain levels in these patients. NMDA receptors include GluN subunits; agonist activity at this level due to increased glutamate modulates the descending pathway at the spinal neuron level. As well as glutamate, glycine (or D-serine) can also act as an agonist activator. NMDA antagonists can block the pain pathway in fibromyalgia through this mechanism.

One study looked at memantine, an NMDA antagonist in fibromyalgia, by measuring metabolite concentrations in the brain using magnetic resonance spectroscopy. Significant increases in N-acetylaspartate and N-acetylaspartate glutamate levels were found in specific areas of the brain. This finding correlated with improved cognition, reduced depression scores and reduced severity of illness at the 3-month follow-up of patients treated with memantine.

One factor for central sensitisation is the wind-up phenomenon; this is the state of progressive increase of responses (temporal summation) induced using repetitive nociceptive stimuli. NMDA antagonists have been found to reduce this wind-up phenomenon and prevent the vicious cycle that causes the persistence of chronic pain in fibromyalgia.

NMDA antagonist preparations and use

Low-dose intravenous ketamine or oral ketamine has been trialled in fibromyalgia syndrome. Ketamine is 2-(2-chlorophenyl)-2-(methylamino)-cyclohexanone and is a non-competitive NMDA antagonist. The S[+] stereoisomer is three to four times more potent than the R[−] isomer. Ketamine also acts on other receptors including muscarinic cholinergic, non-NMDA glutamate, dopaminergic and opioid receptors. Ketamine has significant hallucinogenic properties; it can also cause nausea, headache, dizziness, confusion and psychomimetic effects. In addition, its long-term oral use has been known to cause bladder problems.

Memantine given orally has also been shown to be of benefit. Dextromethorphan given orally has mild NMDA antagonist actions. However, memantine is a non-competitive NMDA antagonist and has been proposed to have a low side-effect profile.

Some studies have used an intravenous dose of 0.2–0.75mg/kg of ketamine or 2mg/kg of oral ketamine. In addition, memantine was used at a dose of 10–30mg/day orally. Long-term use of oral ketamine can cause bladder problems with interstitial cystitis and lower urinary tract symptoms.

Evidence for NMDA antagonists

A recent systematic review found that studies revealed a short-term reduction in pain for a few hours after intravenous infusion of ketamine in patients with fibromyalgia, probably attributable to the nociception-dependent central sensitisation via the NMDA blockade. Case studies showed that the effects lasted longer and were more effective if the total dose was higher and if the infusions were more frequent and of longer duration. The review concluded that there was a dose-response interaction, indicating the potential efficacy of intravenous ketamine in fibromyalgia syndrome.

Another review concluded that the overall benefits of NMDA antagonists in fibromyalgia appeared to be modest. There was a need for better strategy trials to clarify the optimal dose schedules and reduce long-term adverse effects.

A study of 31 patients with fibromyalgia with different treatments showed that ketamine caused a significant reduction in pain intensity during and after the test period. In addition, tender points improved and endurance increased, but the muscle strength was unchanged.

A study of memantine in fibromyalgia found a significant reduction in pain and improved global function, mood and quality of life at 6 months' duration; the NNT was 6.2. Side effects included dizziness and headache.

A randomised double-blinded trial of intravenous infusion of S[+] ketamine in patients with fibromyalgia concluded that the efficacy was limited and restricted in duration; the authors argued that short-term infusion was insufficient to induce long-term analgesic effects in patients with fibromyalgia.

Ketamine given orally has been studied with similarly varied results; a 5-year retrospective study of oral administration followed a trial of intravenous infusion and showed that the pain scores were better in two-thirds of patients, including fewer adverse events. In addition, the results were better in patients who had trialled opioids before.

Most guidelines do not recommend NMDA antagonists in fibromyalgia due to their limited duration of action and the limited evidence. Therefore, a Delphi survey was conducted recently; there was a consensus to evaluate the effectiveness at 1 month and infuse patients with a dose of 0.5–0.9mg/kg/day intravenously for 4 days. The consensus recommended that this treatment be combined with non-pharmacological treatment. They agreed that the risk of adverse events was rare, at less than 3%.

Key Points

- NMDA antagonists can block pain neuromodulation at the glutamate receptor level, preventing wind-up pain and reducing central sensitisation.
- NMDA antagonists have been trialled in many studies, but their actions are short lived, and evidence for them is limited.
- A recent Delphi survey agreed to trial these compounds with non-pharmacological treatment.

References

1. Littlejohn G, Guymer E. Modulation of NMDA receptor activity in fibromyalgia. *Biomedicines* 2017; 5(2): 15.

2. Fayed N, Oliván B, Lopez del Hoyo Y, *et al.* Changes in metabolites in the brain of patients with fibromyalgia after treatment with an NMDA receptor antagonist. *Neuroradiol J* 2019; 32(6): 408-19.

3. Guirimand F, Dupont X, Brasseur L, *et al.* The effects of ketamine on the temporal summation (wind-up) of the R(III) nociceptive flexion reflex and pain in humans. *Anesth Analg* 2000; 90(2): 408-14.

4.   Pastrak M, Abd-Elsayed A, Ma F, *et al.* Systematic review of the use of intravenous ketamine for fibromyalgia. *Ochsner J* 2021; 21(4): 387-94.

5.   Sörensen J, Bengtsson A, Bäckman E, *et al.* Pain analysis in patients with fibromyalgia. Effects of intravenous morphine, lidocaine, and ketamine. *Scand J Rheumatol* 1995; 24(6): 360-5.

6.   Olivan-Blázquez B, Herrera-Mercadal P, Puebla-Guedea M, *et al.* Efficacy of memantine in the treatment of fibromyalgia: a double-blind, randomised, controlled trial with 6-month follow-up. *Pain* 2014; 155(12): 2517-25.

7.   Noppers I, Niesters M, Swartjes M, *et al.* Absence of long-term analgesic effect from a short-term S-ketamine infusion on fibromyalgia pain: a randomized, prospective, double blind, active placebo-controlled trial. *Eur J Pain* 2011; 15(9): 942-9.

8.   Marchetti F, Coutaux A, Bellanger A, *et al.* Efficacy and safety of oral ketamine for the relief of intractable chronic pain: a retrospective 5-year study of 51 patients. *Eur J Pain* 2015; 19(7): 984-93.

9.   Voute M, Riant T, Amodéo JM, *et al.* Ketamine in chronic pain: a Delphi survey. *Eur J Pain* 2022; 26(4): 873-87.

Fibromyalgia

Chapter 47

Cannabinoids

Introduction

Cannabis or marijuana is a psychoactive drug made up of many components: tetrahydrocannabinol (THC), cannabidiol (CBD, hemp), cannabinol (CBN) and tetrahydrocannabivarin. It is the most used illegal drug in the world. Medical use of cannabis is known to reduce chemotherapy-induced nausea, as well as the effects of multiple sclerosis and some resistant forms of epilepsy, but its role in chronic pain and fibromyalgia is debatable.

THC is the main psychoactive component of the cannabis plant. CBD is non-psychotropic.

Nabiximols (Sativex®) is a cannabis extract applied as a spray containing equal ratios of CBD and THC. Dronabinol (THC) and Epidiolex® (CBD) are approved by the United States Food and Drug Administration (US FDA) for anorexia/nausea and rare forms of epilepsy, respectively. Nabilone is a synthetic cannabinoid and mimics THC action.

Mechanism of action

Cannabinoids are highly lipid-soluble and exert action on two types of cannabinoid receptors: CB1 and CB2 receptors, which are G protein-coupled receptors. CB1 is seen mainly in the brain and in some peripheral tissues, whereas CB2 is primarily in peripheral tissues and neuroglial cells.

CB1 receptor agonism can increase dopamine release. Cannabinoid also modulates opioid receptors and potentiates glycine receptors. It also has a 5-HT_{1A} agonist action.

High CBD-to-THC ratios indicate fewer hallucinations and delusional side effects. In addition, CBD has little affinity for cannabinoid receptors.

Cannabis is a Class B controlled drug in the UK. Some states in the USA have legalised the use of cannabis. In Australia, THC was rescheduled recently from S9 (prohibited substances) to S8 (controlled drugs), and licences were granted to permit cannabis cultivation for medicinal use.

Evidence in fibromyalgia

A Cochrane review (2018) concluded that there was no good evidence that any cannabis-derived product works for any chronic neuropathic pain. The review also mentioned that the potential benefits might be outweighed by their potential harm in cases of chronic pain.

Another systematic review also found that the evidence for cannabinoids was of poor quality and concluded that it was unlikely that cannabinoids were highly effective for chronic non-cancer pain.

A few case studies have shown benefits, but these were of low quality and only assessed over the short term. Further research needs to monitor the standardisation of treatment and the evaluation of long-term outcomes, including side effects.

One study looked at adding cannabis-based products to already stable standard analgesic treatments for patients with fibromyalgia; this adjunctive cannabis treatment offered possible advantages for patients, especially those with sleep dysfunction. However, one-third of patients experienced mild adverse events and clinical improvement was correlated inversely with body mass index.

Guidelines

The National Institute for Health and Care Excellence (NICE) recommends NOT to offer any cannabis-based products for chronic pain conditions.

The International Association for the Study of Pain (IASP) has not endorsed the use of cannabinoids in pain due to the lack of evidence; it called for more rigorous and robust research. The IASP is concerned that when the recreational use of cannabis is permitted there is the risk that patients who are experiencing pain could use cannabis without the usual safeguards of medical consultation and monitoring.

The Faculty of Pain Medicine of the Royal College of Anaesthetists, UK, have asserted that cannabis-derived medicinal products' safety and efficacy have not yet been established. It recommended a robust process for developing the evidence for this. The Faculty expressed concern as it viewed potential parallels to the state of high-dose opioids that have had widespread use in the absence of good long-term evidence over the last 20 years and warned and cautioned its members.

The National Academies of Sciences, Engineering, and Medicine (also known as NASEM) warn that although clinical trials have shown a benefit in pain conditions, very little information is known about the efficacy, dose, routes of administration or side effects of commonly used, commercially available cannabis products available in the USA. Furthermore, it clarifies that many cannabis products that are sold in state-regulated markets in the USA bear little resemblance to the products available for research at the federal level.

The Faculty of Pain Medicine of New Zealand and Australia also cautions similarly that the scientific evidence for the efficacy of cannabinoids in the management of chronic pain remains insufficient to justify an endorsement of their clinical use. The Faculty warns and asserts that the sole responsibility of prescribing an unapproved medicinal cannabis product rests with the prescriber.

Self-medication

In a self-reported prevalence study of cannabinoid use in 457 patients with a diagnosis of fibromyalgia in a tertiary pain centre, 13% of patients used cannabinoids; and of these, 80% used herbal cannabis (marijuana), 24% used prescription cannabinoids and 3% used both. Current unstable mental illness (36%), opioid-seeking behaviour (17%) and male sex were associated with herbal cannabis use. The trend that cannabinoid users were unemployed and receiving disability benefits was highlighted. As herbal cannabis use was associated with negative psychosocial parameters, the authors cautioned that any recommendation should be exercised pending clarification of general health and psychosocial problems.

Another large online survey from the USA of 2701 patients with fibromyalgia showed that 60% of patients with fibromyalgia who responded had tried cannabidiol in the past and 32% still used this compound. Among them, 30–40% reported relief across symptom domains.

Purity of CBD oil

CBD is commonly used as an oil orally or by smoking/vaping. The sales of CBD have more than doubled in recent times in the UK. Unlike THC, CBD is legal in the UK and is available as a food product in high street shops and online. A recent report by the British Broadcasting Corporation (BBC) mentioned that half of this type of CBD product contained measurable levels of THC, making them technically illegal. It also found high levels of the solvent dichloromethane in seven products, which could cause respiratory symptoms. Some products did not have the CBD at all, and only 38% of the products tested had CBD levels within 10% of the advertised amount. As it is sold as a food product, there is no legal requirement for these products to be tested.

Key Points

- Cannabinoids exert their actions via the CB1 and CB2 receptors, which are G protein-coupled receptors.
- THC is responsible for psychomimetic actions; a product with a low THC:CBD ratio produces fewer side effects.
- There is a lack of good quality evidence to show that cannabinoids are effective in fibromyalgia.
- NICE recommends NOT to offer any cannabis-based products to treat chronic pain conditions.
- Commercially sold cannabinoids are not regulated and do not contain the promised amount of medication; some have also been found to contain impurities.

References

1. National Institute for Health and Care Excellence; 2021. Cannabis-based medicinal products. NICE guideline NG144. Available from: http://www.nice.org.uk/guidance/ng144.

2. Mücke M, Phillips T, Radbruch L, et al. Cannabis-based medicines for chronic neuropathic pain in adults. Cochrane Database Syst Rev 2018; 3: CD012182.

3. Stockings E, Campbell G, Hall WD, et al. Cannabis and cannabinoids for the treatment of people with chronic non-cancer pain conditions: a systematic review and meta-analysis of controlled and observational studies. Pain 2018; 159(10): 1932-54.

4. Giorgi V, Bongiovanni S, Atzeni F, et al. Adding medical cannabis to standard analgesic treatment for fibromyalgia: a prospective observational study. Clin Exp Rheumatol 2020; 38(1); Suppl 123: 53-9.

5. International Association for the Study of Pain (IASP); 2021. IASP position statement on the use of cannabinoids to treat pain. Available from: https://www.iasp-pain.org/publications/iasp-news/iasp-position-statement-on-the-use-of-cannabinoids-to-treat-pain/.

6. Faculty of Pain Medicine of the Royal College of Anaesthetists; 2021. Update: faculty position statement on the medicinal use of cannabinoids in pain medicine. Available from: https://fpm.ac.uk/update-faculty-position-statement-medicinal-use-cannabinoids-pain-medicine.

7.   Therapeutic effects of cannabis and cannabinoids. In: National Academies of Sciences, Engineering, and Medicine. Washington, DC: National Academies Press; 2017. The health effects of cannabis and cannabinoids: the current state of evidence and recommendations for research. Available from: https://nap.nationalacademies.org/read/24625/chapter/6#89.

8.   Faculty of Pain Medicine ANZCA; 2021. Statement on "Medicinal cannabis" with particular reference to its use in the management of patients with chronic non-cancer pain. Available from: https://www.anzca.edu.au/getattachment/d1eb1074-ef9c-41e6-a1af-31d82b70bcfa/PS10(PM)-Statement-on-Medicinal-Cannabis-with-particular-reference-to-its-use-in-the-management-of-patients-with-chronic-non-cancer-pain.

9.   Ste-Marie PA, Fitzcharles MA, Gamsa A, *et al.* Association of herbal cannabis use with negative psychosocial parameters in patients with fibromyalgia. *Arthritis Care Res* 2012; 64(8): 1202-8.

10.   Boehnke KF, Gagnier JJ, Matallana L, Williams DA. Cannabidiol use for fibromyalgia: prevalence of use and perceptions of effectiveness in a large online survey. *J Pain* 2021; 22(5): 556-66.

11.   Schraer R. BBC; 1 August 2019. CBD oil: have the benefits been overstated? Available from: https://www.bbc.co.uk/news/health-48950483.

Chapter 48

Other medications

Introduction

As discussed in Chapters 5–10, the aetiology of fibromyalgia syndrome is varied; the mechanisms used to change the neuromodulatory pathway and control the symptoms are also varied. Many different medications have been trialled for this condition, but the evidence is limited regarding efficacy and their long-term side effects. This chapter will elaborate on some of these medications and their role in fibromyalgia.

Cyclobenzaprine

Cyclobenzaprine is a centrally acting muscle relaxant acting as a 5-HT$_2$ antagonist and has been used in the USA for fibromyalgia; it is not commonly available in the UK. Side effects include headache, dry mouth, dizziness and arrhythmia. A Cochrane review concluded that there was insufficient evidence to support cyclobenzaprine's use in myofascial pain treatment. The European League Against Rheumatism (EULAR) gave a 'weak for' recommendation for fibromyalgia based on five studies and quoted an NNT of 4.8.

Monoamine oxidase inhibitors (MAOI)

MAOI antidepressants have been trialled in fibromyalgia, but a Cochrane review concluded that their effectiveness was limited. There were data showing some effects on pain and tender points, but these were from small studies with the risk of bias.

Mirogabalin

Mirogabalin is a newer gabapentinoid that has been studied in fibromyalgia; a multicentre study showed that, although mirogabalin showed potential for reducing pain, the primary endpoint of significant pain reduction was not reached when compared with placebo.

Dopamine agonists

The EULAR included recommending dopamine agonists in 2008, but as later trials did not show a benefit, these were not included in the revised 2016 recommendations. In addition, ergoline (partial dopamine agonist) did not improve symptoms in patients with fibromyalgia, except for a subgroup with cervical spinal stenosis.

Growth hormone

Chapter 8 elaborates on the role of growth hormone in the endocrine theory of fibromyalgia. Trials of growth hormone did not show a significant benefit and there were some safety concerns, including sleep apnoea. Therefore, the EULAR strongly recommends against its use in fibromyalgia.

Sodium oxybate

Sodium oxybate is a metabolite of gamma-aminobutyric acid (GABA) and is the sodium salt of gamma-hydroxybutyrate (GHB), an endogenous substance in the brain. It reduces non-restorative sleep abnormalities by improving the quantity and quality of slow-wave sleep. It has been trialled in fibromyalgia. An international phase 3 trial supported evidence that its use provided benefits across multiple symptoms in patients with fibromyalgia. The NNT for 50% pain relief was 5–8. The discontinuation rate was high in this study.

Lacosamide

Lacosamide is an anticonvulsant trialled for fibromyalgia; unfortunately, trials did not show a significant benefit in fibromyalgia.

Key Points

- **Many newer medications have been trialled for fibromyalgia, but the evidence is still limited.**
- **Cyclobenzaprine is a central muscle relaxant with 5-HT$_2$ antagonist action; the EULAR recommends it with weak evidence. It is not commonly available in the UK.**

References

1. Macfarlane GJ, Kronisch C, Dean LE, *et al.* EULAR revised recommendations for the management of fibromyalgia. *Ann Rheum Dis* 2017; 76(2): 318-28.

2. Leite FMG, Atallah AN, El Dib R, *et al.* Cyclobenzaprine for the treatment of myofascial pain in adults. *Cochrane Database Syst Rev* 2009; 3(3): CD006830.

3. Tort S, Urrútia G, Nishishinya MB, Walitt B. Monoamine oxidase inhibitors (MAOIs) for fibromyalgia syndrome. *Cochrane Database Syst Rev* 2012; 4(4): CD009807.

4. Arnold LM, Whitaker S, Hsu C, *et al.* Efficacy and safety of mirogabalin for the treatment of fibromyalgia: results from three 13-week randomized, double-blind, placebo- and active-controlled, parallel-group studies and a 52-week open-label extension study. *Curr Med Res Opin* 2019; 35(10): 1825-35.

5. Distler O, Eich W, Dokoupilova E, *et al.* Evaluation of the efficacy and safety of terguride in patients with fibromyalgia syndrome: results of a twelve-week, multicenter, randomized, double-blind, placebo-controlled, parallel-group study. *Arthritis Rheum* 2010; 62(1): 291-300.

6. Spaeth M, Bennett RM, Benson BA, *et al.* Sodium oxybate therapy provides multidimensional improvement in fibromyalgia: results of an international phase 3 trial. *Ann Rheum Dis* 2012; 71(6): 935-42.

7.   Tzadok R, Ablin JN. Current and emerging pharmacotherapy for fibromyalgia. *Pain Res Manag* 2020;
      2020: ID6541798.

Section 8

Injection therapies

Chapter 49

Intravenous lidocaine infusions

Introduction

Intravenous lidocaine infusions have been used for a long time in patients with fibromyalgia to help ease their symptoms; they play a role in neuromodulation and control of pain and fatigue. However, the evidence is varied and practice differs in different geographical areas.

Mechanism of action

Lidocaine is a local amide anaesthetic; it blocks peripheral and central voltage-gated sodium channels and inhibits ectopic neuronal discharge. A dose of 3–5mg/kg body weight is used intravenously for 1 hour in most centres.

Protocols

Protocols vary in different centres. It is essential to rule out contraindications, including allergy to local anaesthetic and severe cardiac arrhythmia. Usually, a 12-lead electrocardiogram (ECG) is checked and body weight measured. Full monitoring is vital, with blood pressure measured initially more often than every 5 minutes. All resuscitation equipment, including lipid infusion for managing local anaesthetic toxicity, should be available during the procedure.

Variations

Unfortunately, the evidence is limited as there are variations in practice. For example, some centres infuse once every 6 months, while others carry out a series of a few infusions weekly. Depending on local protocols, the dose and way the infusion is given can also vary.

Toxicity

Local anaesthetic toxicity can be fatal if not recognised and treated. The patient can complain of circumoral tingling, followed by tremors, involuntary movements and convulsions. Cardiac signs include abnormal rhythm and low blood pressure. In these circumstances, the infusion should be stopped immediately and resuscitation measures carried out as needed.

Side effects

The above-mentioned fatal effects can take place but are rare. Nevertheless, patients can feel dizzy and light-headed, and should be advised to avoid driving for that day.

Evidence for intravenous lidocaine infusions

A recent systematic review of intravenous lidocaine infusions in patients with fibromyalgia concluded that there was short-term effectiveness and it was safe. However, long-term follow-up has not been studied. Doses between 2 and 7.5mg/kg were used in these studies. The visual analogue score before infusion ranged between 6.1 and 8.1mm, but this improved significantly after treatment to between 1.7 and 4.5mm.

Patients in a study that infused 2–5mg/kg of lidocaine over five daily infusions showed improvement in global impact scores and pain scores after the fifth infusion; these were maintained at 30 days after the fifth infusion.

Another study showed that pain and psychosocial measures improved significantly after intravenous lidocaine infusion in patients with fibromyalgia; the average duration of pain relief was 11.5 weeks in this study. Prospective analysis showed two major (pulmonary oedema and supraventricular tachycardia) and 42 minor side effects out of a total of 106 patients with fibromyalgia receiving the infusion. Nevertheless, 92% of patients found it worthwhile or adequate to try the infusion. The median number of GP (family doctor) visits per month reduced significantly in these patients from 1.5 to 0.5.

Dose-responsiveness

A retrospective analysis of 74 patients with fibromyalgia who had an escalating dose of lidocaine showed that a dose of 7.5mg/kg of lidocaine was safe and had a prolonged effect when compared with the 5mg/kg dose. However, adding 2.5g of magnesium sulfate to the infusion did not benefit significantly.

Toxicity management

If there are signs of toxicity, the lidocaine infusion should be immediately stopped; the usual Airway, Breathing, Circulation, Disability, Exposure (ABC) approach of resuscitation should be applied in the case of toxicity. A call for help immediately is needed as several pairs of hands are required to manage the resuscitation. Airway management with 100% oxygen is vital. If there is a seizure, benzodiazepine, propofol or thiopentone is given in small incremental doses.

Intravenous 20% lipid emulsion is given with an initial bolus of 1.5ml/kg over 1 minute, followed by an infusion of 20% lipid emulsion at 15ml/kg/h. If the patient is not responsive, a maximum of three boluses can be given in total with a 5-minute gap in between; the infusion rate can be doubled to

30ml/kg/h after 5 minutes. The maximum cumulative dose of the 20% lipid emulsion should not exceed 12ml/kg.

Key Points

- Lidocaine infusions cause neuromodulation by blocking voltage-gated sodium channels.
- A dose of 3–5mg/kg body weight infused over 1 hour is commonly practised.
- Full monitoring is vital to rule out cardiac arrhythmias.
- The evidence is variable, but it is commonly practised in many pain centres.
- In cases of toxicity, the ABC approach of resuscitation is applied; administration of a 20% lipid emulsion intravenously is needed.

References

1. de Carvalho JF, Skare TL. Lidocaine in fibromyalgia: a systematic review. *World J Psychiatry* 2022; 12(4): 615-22.

2. Schafranski MD, Malucelli T, Machado F, *et al*. Intravenous lidocaine for fibromyalgia syndrome: an open trial. *Clin Rheumatol* 2009; 28(7): 853-5.

3. Raphael JH, Southall JL, Treharne GJ, Kitas GD. Efficacy and adverse effects of intravenous lignocaine therapy in fibromyalgia syndrome. *BMC Musculoskelet Disord* 2002; 3: 21.

4. Wilderman I, Pugacheva O, Perelman VS, *et al*. Repeated intravenous lidocaine infusions for patients with fibromyalgia: higher doses of lidocaine have a stronger and longer-lasting effect on pain reduction. *Pain Med* 2020; 21(6): 1230-9.

5. AAGBI Safety Guideline: management of severe local anaesthetic toxicity; 2010. Available from: https://anaesthetists.org/Home/Resources-publications/Guidelines/Management-of-severe-local-anaesthetic-toxicity.

Chapter 50

Trigger point injections

Introduction

Trigger point injections are commonly used in myofascial pain syndromes either with a local anaesthetic or with the addition of steroids; pulsed radiofrequency neuromodulation can offer a longer duration of relief if the trigger point injection helps (please refer to Chapter 51 for more detail).

Trigger points

Dr Travell (1942) described the focal 'knots' in a taut band of skeletal muscle as a trigger point. These were described as palpable and caused pain and a local twitch response. Trigger points are different from tender points, which cause local pain, but do not cause referred pain.

In clinical practice, trigger and tender points are used interchangeably and injections are performed in localised painful spots.

Debate on trigger points in fibromyalgia

Fibromyalgia presents with widespread pain; debate always existed on whether modulation of localised trigger points could solve poorly defined generalised symptoms in fibromyalgia. Furthermore, doubts exist on whether these trigger points could be reproduced and identified. Studies have shown some evidence for the efficacy of trigger point injections. In a study on patients with fibromyalgia compared with controls, patients and controls were asked to mark their trigger points and rate their pain. These were quantified using digitisation software. Almost all these trigger points in patients with fibromyalgia were confirmed by a demonstration of spontaneous electrical activity on needle electromyography (EMG).

However, there are inter-clinician reliability issues with identifying taut bands, muscle twitch and active trigger points. Some scientists argue that just like fibrositis and fibrotic nodules have become historical curiosities, trigger points will be eventually discounted as discrete pathological abnormalities in muscle and, instead, myofascial pain will be used widely.

Trigger point injections

In many centres, trigger point injections are carried out as office-based or outpatient procedures. Full asepsis is needed. Ultrasound guidance improves the technical success of these procedures.

Pharmaceutical modelling has proposed that there is a release of algesic substances in muscles and soft tissue in fibromyalgia; these substances can sensitise important nociceptor systems in the pain pathway, including the transient receptor potential vanilloid 1 (TRPV-1) subfamily, acid-sensing ion channel (ASIC) and purinoceptors (P2X3). It has been shown that analgesia in these areas of excessive nociceptive input can provide local as well as general pain relief. The interventions aimed at reducing local fibromyalgia pain have been found to be effective.

Limitations and side effects

Fibromyalgia is a widespread pain affecting many areas of the body. The performance of local trigger point injections might flare up the painful areas in other parts of the body.

The key to managing fibromyalgia is to let the patient take control of their symptom management; trigger points might deviate from this pathway if appropriate education is not given before the procedure. Patients should have explained that injections are not a cure but a way to engage in a multimodal rehabilitation pathway, for which self-management is the key.

Minor rare side effects include infection, bruising and weakness. Allergy to local anaesthetics and/or steroids can be a contraindication. In most centres, if the patient is on long-term anticoagulants, it is wise to continue taking them during the procedure; the risks of bruising are minimal compared with the risks associated with the withdrawal of anticoagulants in these patients.

Evidence for trigger point injections

A systematic review of trigger point injections in chronic non-malignant pain indicated that it was a relatively safe procedure, but there was no clear evidence of either benefit or ineffectiveness of these injections. The study found that adding stretching exercises to trigger point injections augmented the treatment outcomes.

One study compared the efficacy of trigger point injections with botulinum toxin to dry needling and lidocaine in myofascial pain syndromes; it found that local anaesthetic injection was more practical, rapid and cost effective, and was the treatment of choice. If the pain was resistant to conventional treatments, the authors recommend the injection of botulinum toxin.

Another review showed that there is a possible benefit of trigger point injections in effectively reducing pain and increasing pain thresholds in fibromyalgia, based on small randomised controlled trials. This review pointed to the consensus guidelines that concluded support for trigger point injections and their role in the treatment of fibromyalgia.

One study that compared localised muscle or joint injection with placebo showed that an active injection improved fibromyalgia symptoms. It concluded that control of nociceptive input from the somatic periphery enhanced the control of central sensitisation in fibromyalgia syndrome. Pain levels were still low at a 3-week follow-up in the active group of these patients.

A study compared the efficacy of trigger point injections in patients with myofascial pain with or without fibromyalgia. The intervention showed that there was significant improvement in pain parameters and in the range of motion in both groups after 3 weeks. In addition, the range of motion improved immediately in both groups. However, patients with fibromyalgia exhibited delayed and attenuated pain relief after trigger point injection compared with the other group.

Key Points

- Trigger points are focal 'knots' in a taut band of skeletal muscle that causes pain and local twitch responses.
- In common clinical practice, the terms trigger and tender points are used interchangeably, and injections are carried out in painful spots.
- Fibromyalgia presents with widespread pain; trigger point injections should be used together with education regarding self-management as the key.
- Trigger point injections are relatively safe, but there is no clear evidence of their benefit or ineffectiveness.

References

1. Hammi C, Schroeder JD, Yeung B. Trigger point injection. In: StatPearls [Internet]. Treasure Island (FL): StatPearls Publishing; 2021. Available from: https://www.ncbi.nlm.nih.gov/books/NBK542196/.

2. Ge HY, Wang Y, Fernández-de-las-Peñas C, *et al*. Reproduction of overall spontaneous pain pattern by manual stimulation of active myofascial trigger points in fibromyalgia patients. *Arthritis Res Ther* 2011; 13(2): R48.

3.   Bennett RM, Goldenberg DL. Fibromyalgia, myofascial pain, tender points and trigger points: splitting or lumping? *Arthritis Res Ther* 2011; 13(3): 117.

4.   Staud R. Are tender point injections beneficial: the role of tonic nociception in fibromyalgia. *Curr Pharm Des* 2006; 12(1): 23-7.

5.   Scott NA, Guo B, Barton PM, Gerwin RD. Trigger point injections for chronic non-malignant musculoskeletal pain: a systematic review. *Pain Med* 2009; 10(1): 54-69.

6.   Kamanli A, Kaya A, Ardicoglu O, *et al.* Comparison of lidocaine injection, botulinum toxin injection, and dry needling to trigger points in myofascial pain syndrome. *Rheumatol Int* 2005; 25(8): 604-11.

7.   White D, Staff T. Q: do trigger point injections effectively treat fibromyalgia? *J Fam Pract* 2015; 64(7): 427-35.

8.   Affaitati G, Costantini R, Fabrizio A, *et al.* Effects of treatment of peripheral pain generators in fibromyalgia patients. *Eur J Pain* 2011; 15(1): 61-9.

9.   Hong CZ, Hsueh TC. Difference in pain relief after trigger point injections in myofascial pain patients with and without fibromyalgia. *Arch Phys Med Rehabil* 1996; 77(11): 1161-6.

Fibromyalgia

Chapter 51

Pulsed radiofrequency neuromodulation

Introduction

Trigger point injections can be short-lasting; pulsed radiofrequency (PRF) lesions of trigger points and peripheral nerves have been trialled by chronic pain services for more extended pain relief. However, as with trigger points, the evidence base is limited for these procedures.

Pulsed radiofrequency

Pulsed radiofrequency (PRF) is a type of radio wave therapy that aims to reset and modulate the dysfunctional nervous system in fibromyalgia and other chronic pain conditions. Whereas radiofrequency acts by denervating using heat energy, pulsed radiofrequency differs using a lower temperature and causes electrical changes in the nerves; the rapidly changing electrical field is proposed to cause these changes. Therefore, PRF prevents motor nerve lesioning and is considered safer. A popular theory for the pulsed radiofrequency mechanism is that it causes neuromodulation by altering the pain pathway via c-fos, an immediate-early gene involved in transmission. Increased c-fos expression was seen in animal experiments in dorsal root ganglia pulsed radiofrequency application. This mechanism can inhibit the excitatory C-fibres and cause long-term depression in nerve conduction. c-fos gene expression can lead to modulation of the endogenous endorphin pathway.

Applications

PRF is delivered using a specific machine via standard needles. It uses radiofrequency current in short 20-millisecond high voltage bursts; this is followed by a silent phase of 480 milliseconds that allows heat to be dissipated, thereby keeping the tissue temperature at less than 42°C.

Practicalities

PRF can be applied on trigger points or in peripheral nerves. Ultrasound guidance is often used to aid needle direction and visualisation before injections. The use of sterile areas and universal precautions for sterilisation are vital. The benefits can last from 6–9 months.

Evidence for PRF

Scientific evidence on PRF in patients with fibromyalgia is limited to case reports only; many of these studies include a wide variety of pain conditions, including fibromyalgia. For example, a series of trials of PRF in different types of pain, including fibromyalgia, showed that 67% of patients had pain relief for more than 6 months, and a few had more than 1-year relief.

Key Points

- PRF can prolong the benefits of trigger point injections.
- PRF keeps tissue temperature to less than 42°C; it spares motor nerves and is safe.
- The evidence on PRF is limited to case reports only.

References

1.   Byrd D, Mackey S. Pulsed radiofrequency for chronic pain. *Curr Pain Headache Rep* 2008; 12(1): 37-41.

2.   Van Zundert J, de Louw AJ, Joosten EAJ, *et al.* Pulsed and continuous radiofrequency current adjacent to the cervical dorsal root ganglion of the rat induces late cellular activity in the dorsal horn. *Anesthesiology* 2005; 102(1): 125-31.

3.   Al Tamimi M, McCeney MH, Krutsch J. A case series of pulsed radio frequency treatment of myofascial trigger points and scar neuromas. *Pain Med* 2009; 20(6): 1140-3.

Fibromyalgia

Chapter 52

Infusions of other medications

Introduction

Apart from intravenous lidocaine infusion, various other pharmacological agents have been trialled by infusion with limited evidence. This chapter will detail a few of these chemicals used in patients with fibromyalgia.

These agents are given intravenously and can have potential side effects. They need to be used with appropriate monitoring and resuscitation facilities; discharge from the day-case area should be done after appropriate recovery protocols.

Intravenous magnesium

Magnesium infusion has been used for various conditions, including arrhythmias, resistant asthma, eclampsia and hypomagnesaemia. In addition, it has been trialled in patients with fibromyalgia alone or in combination with lidocaine infusion.

Magnesium can act as a smooth muscle relaxant by blocking calcium channels. In addition, it is an antagonist for the N-methyl-D-aspartate (NMDA) receptor, which could explain its effects on chronic pain modulation and attenuation of central sensitisation.

A systematic review of intravenous magnesium in various pain conditions concluded that the evidence for the efficacy is globally modest with a limited number of studies.

A retrospective review of infusion therapies in fibromyalgia showed a trend of greater response to 2.5g of magnesium sulphate as an adjunct to intravenous lidocaine infusion, but without statistical significance. A combination of lidocaine and magnesium infusions reduced the pain scores by 2.41–3.62 on average, which corresponded to 30.51–46.71% in the short term; in the long term, administration gave an average pain relief of 30.23–40.68%.

Intravenous ketamine

Ketamine is an NMDA receptor antagonist; it reduces glutamatergic synaptic transmission in the spinal cord and brain. This change leads to a reduction in synaptic plasticity and decreases the maintenance of the chronic pain state in fibromyalgia. Studies have used doses of 0.3–0.5mg/kg over 30 minutes as an infusion.

Side effects include nausea, dizziness, hallucinations, confusion and drowsiness; usually, these are short-lived.

A systematic review of intravenous ketamine in fibromyalgia showed a dose-response potential efficacy. Longer periods of more frequent infusions may be associated with more effective and longer-lasting analgesic relief.

A double-blinded, placebo-controlled study of patients with fibromyalgia showed a significant reduction in pain intensity scores that lasted 2–7 days after a single infusion of 0.3mg/kg of ketamine. In addition, significant decreases in tender points and improved muscle endurance were noted in these patients.

A higher dose infusion case report was found to give long-term pain relief for more than a year with improved quality of life. A dose of 200–800mg infused over 4 hours for 5 days, followed by a booster of 800mg at 2 weeks, gave longer relief for this patient with fibromyalgia.

Other intravenous infusions

Various other intravenous infusions have been trialled in chronic pain states such as fibromyalgia without proven evidence; these case reports include:

- Dexmedetomidine: selective alpha-2 adrenergic agonist that binds to transmembrane G protein-binding adrenoceptors; infusion can help in widespread pain. Side effects include hypotension, bradycardia and respiratory depression.
- Clonidine: selective alpha-2 adrenergic agonist with actions similar to that of dexmedetomidine.
- Phentolamine: alpha-2 adrenergic antagonist that has been trialled for chronic pain with side effects of hypotension, tachycardia and gastrointestinal upset.

Key Points

- Intravenous magnesium acts by calcium channel blockade and antagonistic action at NMDA receptors.
- Magnesium has been trialled and given intravenously, but the evidence is still limited.
- Intravenous ketamine acts as an antagonist to NMDA receptors.
- Other infusions have been trialled and documented in case reports with no evidence at present.
- An infusion of chemicals can help in resistant symptom presentation in fibromyalgia.

References

1.   Morel V, Pickering ME, Goubayon J, *et al.* Magnesium for pain treatment in 2021? State of the art. *Nutrients* 2021; 13(5): 1397.

2.   Wilderman I, Pugacheva O, Perelman VS, *et al.* Repeated intravenous lidocaine infusions for patients with fibromyalgia: higher doses of lidocaine have a stronger and longer-lasting effect on pain reduction. *Pain Med* 2020; 21(6): 1230-9.

3.   Pastrak M, Abd-Elsayed A, Ma F, *et al.* Systematic review of the use of intravenous ketamine for fibromyalgia. *Ochsner J* 2021; 21(4): 387-94.

4.   Sörensen J, Bengtsson A, Bäckman E, *et al.* Pain analysis in patients with fibromyalgia: effects of intravenous morphine, lidocaine, and ketamine. *Scand J Rheumatol* 1995; 24(6): 360-5.

5.   Hanna AF, Smith AJ. Intravenous ketamine produces long-term pain relief in a patient with fibromyalgia. *Fibrom Open Access* 2016; 1(1): 104.

6.   Kosharskyy B, Almonte W, Shaparin N, *et al.* Intravenous infusions in chronic pain management. *Pain Phys* 2013; 16(3): 231-49.

Chapter 53

Other injections

Introduction

Nerve blocks are common interventions used in rehabilitating patients with chronic pain conditions such as fibromyalgia. They help break the vicious cycle of pain, stiffness and reduced activity; they encourage patients by giving them the confidence to engage in physiotherapy and their supported self-management pathway.

Essentialities

Education must precede any intervention in patients with fibromyalgia. Patients should be advised about exercise and pacing strategies; the need to keep active by gradual activities should be emphasised before they are listed for injection procedures. During and after the injection treatment, the most important and relevant points should be stressed again so that injections are used as part of a multimodal management pathway in rehabilitation.

Practicalities

Most of these procedures are carried out as outpatient or office-based procedures. Universal sterile precautions are vital to prevent infection-related complications. It is wise to avoid steroids if possible and use local anaesthetic injections, followed by pulsed radiofrequency if feasible later.

Peripheral nerve blocks

Many pain services offer a variety of peripheral nerve blocks with the sole aim of giving pain relief in the short term to help the patients engage in physiotherapy and gradual mobilisation. Ultrasound-guided peripheral nerve blocks are practised routinely in most pain centres.

Greater occipital nerve blocks

Headaches are a common presentation in patients with fibromyalgia; they can significantly affect the quality of life of these patients. Therefore, pain clinics commonly use bilateral greater occipital nerve blocks under ultrasound guidance to help ease this pain.

Botulinum toxin injections for headache

Botulinum toxin injections are used to relieve migraine headaches in patients with fibromyalgia. The toxin is extracted from the anaerobic bacterium *Clostridium botulinum*, with seven of its 40 subtypes showing antigen specificity. The toxin is organised as a double-chain protein, with the light chain being the active form. Botulinum toxin type A (BoNT-A) and type B (BoNT-B) are commonly used in pain medicine.

At the neuromuscular junction, a complex of soluble N-ethylmaleimide-sensitive factor attachment protein receptor (SNARE) proteins, including syntaxin, synaptobrevin and synaptosomal-associated protein 25 (SNAP-25), are involved in the release of acetylcholine, resulting in muscle contractions. Botulinum toxin blocks the presynaptic release of acetylcholine at the neuromuscular junction by breaking down this SNARE protein complex, causing muscle relaxation, which leads to its analgesic effects. In addition, this process also releases neuropeptides, such as substance P and calcitonin gene-related peptide (CGRP), in nociceptive neurons, contributing to analgesia.

The National Institute for Health and Care Excellence (NICE), in its technology appraisal guidance, has recommended BoNT-A for chronic migraine prophylaxis in patients suffering from headaches for at least 15 days every month and who have not responded to at least three medications. If patients show improved headache symptoms, BoNT-A can be continued. However, it should be discontinued if patients show less than 30% symptomatic relief after two injections. As per the NICE guidelines, Botox® is injected in 31 sites or more, at a dose of 5 units for each site, with a maximum of 200 units.

Suprascapular nerve blocks

Suprascapular nerve blocks relieve shoulder pain if this is the worst focus of pain in patients with fibromyalgia. In addition, ultrasound-guided diagnostic local anaesthetic injection followed by pulsed radiofrequency is routinely used in many pain centres.

Limitations of injections in fibromyalgia

In patients with fibromyalgia with widespread dysaesthesia, reducing local pain in one area can flare up other pain. This outcome should be explained and informed during the consent process. A selective minimalistic interventional trial followed by pulsed radiofrequency can limit these complications.

Patients should be informed to take control of their pain rather than have a passive dependence on these injections. Long-term relief depends on appropriate education with engagement in gradual pacing strategies to mobilise, using injections as a tool to achieve this goal.

Key Points

- Various peripheral injection interventions are used in patients with fibromyalgia to ease pain and engage in recovery.
- Injections have limitations and should be used to harness the benefit to engage in multimodal recovery.
- Greater occipital blocks and botulinum toxin injections are used in fibromyalgia for patients with headaches.

References

1. Vasu T. Nerve blocks. In: Vasu T. *Managing long COVID syndrome*. Shrewsbury, UK: tfm publishing Ltd; 2022: pp. 259-62.
2. Vasu T. Botox treatment for headache. In: Vasu T. *Managing long COVID syndrome*. Shrewsbury, UK: tfm publishing Ltd; 2022: pp. 263-6.

Section 9

Psychological therapies

Fibromyalgia

Chapter 54

Psychology

Introduction

Comprehensive multidisciplinary pain management services include psychology and value its role in self-management strategies to aid recovery in fibromyalgia syndrome. A low mood, frustration, anxiety and a state of helplessness are commonly encountered in patients with fibromyalgia. The outcomes from fibromyalgia are poorer in patients with low mood and depression.

Education and explanation play a major role in the outcome of these patients. Good communication skills also play a great role in helping these patients with fibromyalgia understand the need to avoid irrational fears.

Pain catastrophising

'Pain catastrophising' is a commonly used term in pain clinics; 'catastrophising' is an exaggerated fear of pain or pain experience. It is associated with a lack of confidence and control and leads to poor outcomes.

Psychological flexibility

Psychological flexibility relates to being in contact with the present moment, fully aware of emotions, sensations and thoughts, welcoming them, including the undesired ones, and moving towards behaviour of chosen values. Studies have shown that psychological flexibility correlates with improved outcomes in patients with fibromyalgia. Acceptance and commitment therapy (ACT) uses psychological flexibility to modulate human adaptation and well-being.

Fear avoidance

The fear-avoidance theory is popularly used in pain services to explain why fear can cause limited mobility, disengagement with activity and lead to disuse. Normally, after injury, we manage our fears, confront them and recover; in susceptible patients, the pain experience and fear can lead to a vicious cycle and cause persistent pain.

Sleep and mood

Sleep interruption and poor sleep hygiene play a major role in the persistence of chronic pain and fatigue in fibromyalgia. Therefore, education regarding sleep hygiene is a vital component of the chronic pain management plan. Furthermore, medications for pain can cause poor-quality sleep. Please refer to Chapter 59 for more details on sleep management in fibromyalgia.

Yellow flags

Yellow flags are psychosocial factors that are indicative of long-term chronicity and disability. These include a negative attitude that pain is harmful and disabling, fear avoidance and reduced activity, an expectation of passive treatments, a tendency for depression and social withdrawal, and social/financial problems.

It is important to address these issues right at the beginning of the rehabilitation pathway in fibromyalgia; this helps to ensure that appropriate care is given and appropriate actions are taken to prevent chronicity. Addressing these issues, however, is more difficult in fibromyalgia syndrome, given that this illness has devastating effects on the social, financial and psychological aspects of patients' lives.

Pathophysiological changes

Fibromyalgia and depression are specific syndromes with their own proposed pathophysiological changes in the central nervous system. In both conditions, physical and psychological stress can change the hypothalamic-pituitary-adrenal (HPA) axis (please refer to Chapters 6 and 8 for more detail). These changes can activate the serotonergic system via the amygdala and raphe nuclei. Noradrenergic system activation occurs via the locus coeruleus in the rostral pons of the brain; the locus coeruleus is involved in the stress response, arousal and sleep, and it projects towards the hypothalamus. All these changes lead to modulation in the prefrontal cortex area. The HPA axis is involved in memory and learning related to the pain experience.

Diathesis-stress theory

Although the diathesis-stress model is commonly used in mental health illnesses, it could also easily be applied to fibromyalgia syndrome. This psychological theory explains that people with particular vulnerabilities respond differently to stress than others. While most patients with particular tendencies can self-regulate their mood and cognitions in response to stress, patients with fibromyalgia have tendencies that do not allow them to cope with a challenge and become vulnerable to depression. In summary, the link between a particular environment (stressors) and particular tendencies can make patients prone to a response output with symptoms of fibromyalgia syndrome.

Assessing and measuring mood in chronic pain

The Hospital Anxiety and Depression Scale (HADS) has been commonly used in many pain services to score anxiety and depression levels. It is easy to score and is based on how the patients felt the previous week. A score of

8–10 is considered borderline; a score of more than 11 needs to be monitored and treated appropriately.

Various other scores have been used to assess the psychological status of a patient. Each pain service uses its preferred sets of scores to look at diagnosis, treatment pathway and management. It helps to assess outcomes in terms of quality-of-life improvement of patients.

Other scores include:

- Brief Pain Inventory (BPI).
- EuroQol score for quality assessment in various dimensions (EQ-5D).
- Pain Anxiety Symptoms Scale (PASS).
- Survey of Pain Attitudes (SOPA).
- Chronic Pain Coping Inventory (CPCI).
- Chronic Pain Acceptance Questionnaire (CPAQ).
- Pain Catastrophising Scale (PCS).

Coping strategies and pain

A study of patients with fibromyalgia concluded using multilevel analyses that higher pain levels in patients with an uncertainty of illness predicted difficulties in coping mechanisms.

Depression and fibromyalgia

Both depression and fibromyalgia have similar pathophysiology: similar predisposing, precipitating and perpetuating factors. Both are targeted by similar drugs acting on serotoninergic and noradrenergic systems. Both conditions have a similar genetic predisposition and environmental stressor or triggering event.

One study compared patients with neuropathic pain and those with fibromyalgia pain. Although both groups had similar pain intensities, the incidence of depression per the diagnostic criteria was significantly higher in fibromyalgia syndrome (7.1%) compared with neuropathic pain (3.3%).

A systematic review showed that patients with fibromyalgia and comorbid depression had poorer outcomes of multimodal rehabilitation than patients with fibromyalgia without depression. Those with depression had more sleep disturbances, sexual dysfunction, loss of physical function level and a lower quality of life. It is vital that the clinician tries to explore this aspect in their consultation and motivates these patients to seek therapy with the aim of seeking support in coping with depression.

Anxiety and fibromyalgia

A study looked at a structured clinical interview for the Diagnostic and Statistical Manual for Mental Disorders (DSM-IV) in patients with fibromyalgia. It concluded that fibromyalgia is not a homogeneous diagnosis, but shows varying proportions of comorbid anxiety and depression, depending on the psychosocial characteristics of the patients. It stressed the need to treat both the physical and emotional domains of fibromyalgia syndrome.

Catastrophising in fibromyalgia

A prominent feature in fibromyalgia is the irrational or exaggerated fear of the pain experience. One study showed that, compared with other chronic pain conditions such as rheumatoid arthritis, patients with fibromyalgia have a more pronounced link between catastrophising and self-reported pain. This finding indicates that treating pain and depression together is essential in patients with fibromyalgia; cognitive therapy and coping skills are essential to any comprehensive management programme for fibromyalgia.

Fibromyalgia-specific scoring systems

The Fibromyalgia Impact Questionnaire (FIQ) is used in many research projects. The FIQ measures physical functioning, work status, depression, anxiety, morning tiredness, pain, stiffness, fatigue and well-being over the previous week. The revised 2009 version consists of 21 items across three domains of function (n = 9), overall impact (n = 2) and symptoms (n = 10). It is a self-administered questionnaire and takes approximately 5 minutes to complete.

Talking therapies

All pain services offer some form of talking therapy; self-referral schemes might also be available in the community. Some forms of talking therapy may include:

- Cognitive behavioural therapy (CBT).
- Improving Access to Psychological Therapies (IAPT), an NHS initiative to improve mental health.
- Psychodynamic therapy.
- Group therapy.
- Counselling.
- Next-generation psychological therapies.

Cognitive behavioural therapy

CBT has been found effective in providing coping strategies for patients with fibromyalgia. CBT helps to manage mental illness by changing how a patient thinks (cognition) and behaves (behaviour), so they can change how they feel. Thoughts, feelings and actions are interrelated, and negative thinking can result in a patient being caught in a vicious cycle. The role of CBT is to explore these interlinks and address the problem by changing the patient's negative thinking pattern. In addition, it helps the patient break down the problems of fibromyalgia syndrome into smaller chunks, so they gain confidence in dealing and coping with the problem positively.

CBT aims to identify challenging, unhelpful thoughts in patients with fibromyalgia syndrome. Once identified, the patient is taken through a graded exposure, reducing unhelpful behaviours and removing unnecessary fears. Please refer to Chapter 55 for more details.

Acceptance and commitment therapy

Whereas CBT teaches patients how to control their thoughts, feelings and memories, acceptance and commitment therapy (ACT) involves the patient with fibromyalgia in accepting and embracing their problem and committing to their recovery from these difficulties. ACT is based on the relational frame theory, which proposes that rational skills may not be effective when faced with a psychological problem and teaches the patient to accept the problem as normal and learn ways to live more healthily. In addition, it uses mindfulness-based approaches that are discussed in the following paragraphs. The use of metaphors is common in ACT to engage the patient with fibromyalgia in the acceptance pathway.

ACT focuses on the patient embracing their thoughts and feelings, leading to a commitment to recovery and behavioural changes. Although it may not necessarily help the patient accept the sequelae of fibromyalgia syndrome, it will help them accept the unwanted experiences suffered as a consequence of the condition. Please refer to Chapter 56 for more details.

The six core principles of ACT that help to develop psychological flexibility include:

- Cognitive defusion.
- Acceptance.
- Being in the present moment.
- Self as context.
- Discovering values.
- Committed action.

Mindfulness-based approaches

Mindfulness focuses on the present moment rather than dwelling on the multiple problems and catastrophising. It helps the patient with fibromyalgia to be fully aware of where they are and what they are doing and not to be overwhelmed by what happens outside.

In a patient with fibromyalgia, this approach uses meditation techniques that help the patient live in, and concentrate on, the present moment, using any of the senses, including touch, sight, sound, taste or smell. Therefore, mindfulness creates awareness of thoughts in the present moment.

Mindfulness-based stress reduction and mindfulness-based cognitive therapy may have a significant role in the rehabilitation pathway for patients with fibromyalgia syndrome if incorporated as part of multimodal treatment. Please refer to Chapter 57 for more details.

Comparison of various psychological therapies

A meta-analysis looking at various psychological interventions in fibromyalgia showed small-to-medium pain reduction in the long term over an average follow-up of 7.4 months. They also improved sleep, depression, functional status and catastrophising. This review concluded that cognitive behavioural treatment is significantly better than other psychological treatments in short-term pain reduction. In addition, higher treatment doses were associated with better outcomes.

A randomised trial comparing multicomponent CBT with or without hypnosis and pharmacological treatment showed that CBT had better outcomes than pharmacological treatment. The addition of hypnosis enhanced the effectiveness of the psychological treatment.

Evidence for psychological therapies

A Cochrane review suggested that psychological therapies may be effective in improving physical functioning, pain and low mood for adults with fibromyalgia, but the quality of evidence was low.

Complexities in the psychological management of fibromyalgia

A patient with fibromyalgia can face significant problems with identity and core integrity, as many healthcare professionals do not understand the complex pathophysiology and can question the legitimacy of symptoms and their diagnosis. Furthermore, the coping strategy of an individual is deeply embedded in their social situation, varying with their health identity, socioeconomic situation, age, gender, ethnicity, religion and disability.

Illness intrusiveness includes the disruption of patients' valued activities, lifestyle and interests, which can compromise their quality of life. Illness-induced disruption can interfere with the results of treatment including its side effects and complications; it can also impact the state of health of the affected person.

Key Points

- Psychology has an important role in managing fibromyalgia syndrome; it should be a part of the multimodal management pathway.
- 'Catastrophising' is an exaggerated irrational fear of pain.
- Fear avoidance leads to a vicious cycle of reduced mobility and exaggerated pain.
- Yellow flags are psychosocial factors that indicate chronicity in fibromyalgia.
- Depression is more common in patients with fibromyalgia than in other chronic pain conditions.
- CBT, ACT and mindfulness-based approaches are commonly used in combination with other treatments for fibromyalgia.

References

1.   Vasu T. Psychology in chronic pain. In: Vasu T, Balasubramanian S, Kodivalasa M, Ingle PM, Eds. *Chronic pain management*. Shrewsbury, UK: tfm publishing Ltd; 2021: pp. 183-7.

2.   Ramaci T, Bellini D, Presti G, Santisi G. Psychological flexibility and mindfulness as predictors of individual outcomes in hospital health workers. *Front Psychol* 2019; 10: 1302.

3.   Thiagarajah AS, Guymer EK, Leech M, Littlejohn GO. The relationship between fibromyalgia, stress and depression. *Int J Clin Rheumatol* 2014; 9(4): 371-84.

4.   Johnson LM, Zautra AJ, Davis MC. The role of illness uncertainty on coping with fibromyalgia symptoms. *Health Psychol* 2006; 25(6): 696-703.

5.   Gracely RH, Ceko M, Bushnell MC. Fibromyalgia and depression. *Pain Res Treat* 2012; 2012: 486590.

6.   Gormsen L, Rosenberg R, Bach FW, Jensen TS. Depression, anxiety, health-related quality of life and pain in patients with chronic fibromyalgia and neuropathic pain. *Eur J Pain* 2010; 14(2): 127.e1-8.

7.   Lange M, Petermann F. Influence of depression on fibromyalgia: a systematic review. *Schmerz* 2010; 24(4): 326-33.

8.   Thieme K, Turk DC, Flor H. Comorbid depression and anxiety in fibromyalgia syndrome: relationship to somatic and psychosocial variables. *Psychosom Med* 2004; 66(6): 837-44.

9.   Hassett AL, Cone JD, Patella SJ, Sigal LH. The role of catastrophizing in the pain and depression of women with fibromyalgia syndrome. *Arthritis Rheum* 2000; 43(11): 2493-500.

10.   American College of Rheumatology. Fibromyalgia Impact Questionnaire. Available from: https://www.rheumatology.org/I-Am-A/Rheumatologist/Research/Clinician-Researchers/Fibromyalgia-Impact-Questionnaire-FIQ.

11.   Glombiewski JA, Sawyer AT, Gutermann J, *et al.* Psychological treatments for fibromyalgia: a meta-analysis. *Pain* 2010; 151(2): 280-95.

12.   Castel A, Cascón R, Padrol A, *et al.* Multicomponent cognitive-behavioral group therapy with hypnosis for the treatment of fibromyalgia: long-term outcome. *J Pain* 2012; 13(3): 255-65.

13.   Theadom A, Cropley M, Smith HE, *et al.* Mind and body therapy for fibromyalgia. *Cochrane Database Syst Rev* 2015; 4(4): CD001980.

14.   Lempp HK, Hatch SL, Carville SF, Choy EH. Patients' experiences of living with and receiving treatment for fibromyalgia syndrome: a qualitative study. *BMC Musculoskelet Disord* 2009; 10: 124.

Chapter 55

Cognitive behavioural therapies

Introduction

Cognitive behavioural therapies (CBTs) help manage the way a patient thinks (cognition) and behaves (behaviour) so that they can change the way they feel.

Thoughts, feelings and actions are interrelated (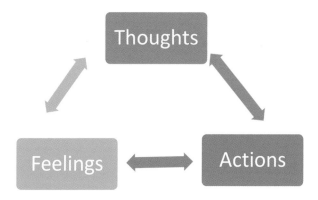 Figure 55.1). Negative thinking can result in patients with fibromyalgia being caught in a vicious

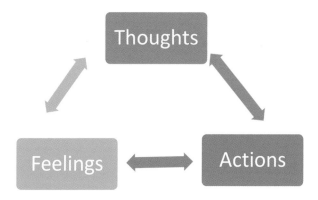

Figure 55.1. Thoughts, feelings and actions.

cycle of low mood, inactivity and worsening pain. CBT explores these interlinks and addresses the problem by changing the negative thinking pattern in a patient with fibromyalgia.

CBT practicalities

CBT guides the patient with fibromyalgia to break down the problems into smaller chunks, helping the patient gain confidence in dealing and coping positively.

To achieve this, the therapist will facilitate the patient to identify challenging and unhelpful thoughts. Once patients realise these thoughts and the impact on their life, they are motivated to look at ways of dealing with them.

Graded exposure to reduce these unhelpful behaviours will lead to a pathway of recovery and remove unnecessary fears.

Neurophysiology of CBT

Catastrophising is correlated with increased resting-state functional connectivity between the S1 area (primary somatosensory cortex) and the anterior insula in the brain. One study used resting-state fMRI (rs-fMRI) scans to evaluate functional connectivity. It showed that CBT led to greater reductions in catastrophising-related rs-fMRI changes compared with a control group. Furthermore, both pain and catastrophising were reduced significantly at a 6-month follow-up in this study.

Evidence for CBT in fibromyalgia

A Cochrane review of CBT in patients with fibromyalgia concluded that there was a small incremental benefit over a control group in reducing pain, negative mood and disability at the end of the treatment and long-term follow-up.

A systematic review of CBT in patients with fibromyalgia syndrome showed no significant effect on pain, fatigue, sleep and health-related quality of life (HRQoL), but it improved mood problems after therapy. In addition, it concluded that CBT could improve coping strategies and reduce the depressed mood and healthcare-seeking behaviour in fibromyalgia.

A randomised clinical trial compared sessions of a cognitive therapy group with group discussion alone and people on the waiting list. It was shown that the 12-session cognitive treatment group did not improve outcomes compared with group education and discussion. The short-term success rate was 6.4% for the cognitive group and 18.4% for group discussion.

The authors concluded that the fear reduction had enhanced pain coping and control through group education, whereas poor compliance, the difficulty with homework assignments and the lack of individual support had limited the effectiveness of the cognitive treatment group. The economic evaluation showed that adding a cognitive component to the educational intervention led to significantly higher healthcare costs and no additional improvement in quality of life.

An interdisciplinary consensus guideline stated that isolated CBT in patients with fibromyalgia does not show clear benefits over group programmes of education or exercise. However, it concluded with recommendations that CBT was effective in specific subgroups with higher psychosocial malaise.

A randomised trial of multidisciplinary treatments in fibromyalgia with or without CBT showed that CBT mildly increased the effect of the outcome benefits in patients with fatigue.

Online CBT for fibromyalgia

A 6-week online internet-based CBT showed benefits of a lower fibromyalgia impact score and lower tender point scores at 6- and 12-week follow-up in a small group of patients with fibromyalgia. However, these were low-quality studies reviewed only for the short term. The COVID pandemic has led to many CBT and pain management programmes being carried out online, and the results of these evaluations are awaited.

Guidelines

Recent NICE guidelines for chronic primary pain recommend that CBT be delivered by healthcare professionals with appropriate training.

The European League Against Rheumatism (EULAR) gives a weak recommendation for supporting CBT in patients with fibromyalgia. It looked at five reviews and up to 30 trials to come to this conclusion.

Limitations of CBT

Patients with fibromyalgia might have negative emotions, including anger towards themselves. The way these patients process and regulate these emotions can be relevant to amplifying their pain output. Behaviour therapies such as CBT use cognitive restructuring, which can have less impact on patients with fibromyalgia who score highly in the intensity of the affect. However, results from CBT in fibromyalgia are limited in the long term.

Key Points

- CBT changes the way patients think and behave to change how they feel.
- The evidence is variable for CBT in fibromyalgia.
- A Cochrane review quotes a small incremental benefit for CBT in patients with fibromyalgia.
- NICE guidelines recommend CBT for chronic primary pain if delivered by appropriately trained clinicians.

References

1. Vasu T. Psychology in chronic pain. In: Vasu T, Balasubramanian S, Kodivalasa M, Ingle PM, Eds. *Chronic pain management*. Shrewsbury, UK: tfm publishing Ltd; 2021: pp. 183-7.

2. Lazaridou A, Kim J, Cahalan CM, *et al*. Effects of cognitive-behavioral therapy (CBT) on brain connectivity supporting catastrophizing in fibromyalgia. *Clin J Pain* 2017; 33(3): 215-21.

3. Bernardy K, Klose P, Busch AJ, *et al*. Cognitive behavioural therapies for fibromyalgia. *Cochrane Database Syst Rev* 2013; 9(9): CD009796.

4. Bernardy K, Füber N, Köllner V, Häuser W. Efficacy of cognitive-behavioral therapies in fibromyalgia syndrome – a systematic review and metaanalysis of randomized controlled trials. *J Rheumatol* 2010; 37(10): 1991-2005.

5. Vlaeyen JW, Teeken-Gruben NJ, Goossens ME, *et al*. Cognitive-educational treatment of fibromyalgia: a randomized clinical trial. I. Clinical effects. *J Rheumatol* 1996; 23(7): 1237-45.

6. Goossens ME, Rutten-van Mölken MP, Leidl RM, *et al*. Cognitive-educational treatment of fibromyalgia: a randomized clinical trial. II. Economic evaluation. *J Rheumatol* 1996; 23(7): 1246-54.

7. De Miquel CA, Campayo JG, Flórez MT, *et al*. Interdisciplinary consensus document for the treatment of fibromyalgia. *Actas Esp Psiquiatr* 2010; 38(2): 108-20.

8. Lera S, Gelman SM, López MJ, *et al*. Multidisciplinary treatment of fibromyalgia: does cognitive behavior therapy increase the response to treatment? *J Psychosom Res* 2009; 67(5): 433-41.

9. Menga G, Ing S, Khan O, *et al*. Fibromyalgia: can online cognitive behavioral therapy help? *Ochsner J* 2014; 14(3): 343-9.

10. Amutio A, Franco C, de Carmen Perez-Fuentes M, *et al*. Mindfulness training for reducing anger, anxiety, and depression in fibromyalgia patients. *Front Psychol* 2015; 5: 1572.

11. National Institute for Health and Care Excellence; 2021. Chronic pain (primary and secondary) in over 16s: assessment of all chronic pain and management of chronic primary pain. NICE guideline, NG193. Available from: http://www.nice.org.uk/guidance/ng193/chapter/recommendations.

12. Macfarlane GJ, Kronisch C, Dean LE, *et al*. EULAR revised recommendations for the management of fibromyalgia. *Ann Rheum Dis* 2017; 76(2): 318-28.

Fibromyalgia

Chapter 56

Acceptance and commitment therapies

Introduction

Whereas the previous generation of psychological therapies looked at ways to control thoughts, feelings and memories, acceptance and commitment therapy (ACT) looks at how a patient with fibromyalgia could accept and embrace the problem and commit to the recovery pathway.

ACT and practicalities

ACT is based on the relational frame theory. This theory proposes that rational skills may not be effective when a patient is faced with a psychological problem. It teaches how to live healthily by accepting the problem. ACT focuses on functioning rather than symptom reduction in a patient with fibromyalgia.

Acceptance does not mean that the patient must accept the sequelae of the fibromyalgia syndrome; it just focuses on how to accept the unwanted experiences suffered as a result of the condition.

Relational frame theory

The response to any stimulus changes based on our learning and experiences; they are guided by contextual cues, relating themselves to others.

The environment plays a bigger role in how the response occurs to a stimulus. Undoing a relational context might not be possible, but focusing and training on its functional context can lead to better outcomes. ACT trains the patient with fibromyalgia to experience the same thought without negatively affecting the action while allowing the content of the thought to stay as before.

Functional contextualism

ACT is based on a philosophical framework called functional contextualism; this is based on two concepts:

- Chosen unit of analysis: looking at the whole event; formally, similar actions might have different functions depending on the context. None of the experiences is inherently problematic or positive; it depends on how they function for that person at that time.
- Truth criterion: effective action; refining the general criterion to a more specific goal. This will help to achieve a meaningful clinical goal or outcome.

ACT takes the cognition out of the way so the patient with fibromyalgia can interact with the actual contingencies.

Components of ACT

The six core principles of ACT that help to develop psychological flexibility include:

- Cognitive defusion.
- Acceptance.
- Being in the present moment.
- Self as context.
- Discovering values.
- Committed action.

Use of metaphors

ACT practitioners use metaphors, stories, role plays and exercises to help patients understand the complexity of the pathophysiology of fibromyalgia and develop psychological flexibility. Commonly used metaphors in clinical practice in fibromyalgia include a bus driver with disturbing passengers (with the focus on accepting and committing to the drive), a tug of war with a monster (to let go and accept rather than be afraid of the monster), a sailing boat with a hole (rather than bailing out water, the need to focus on the direction) and demons on the boat (a focus on where to direct the boat and accept the demons).

Evidence for ACT in fibromyalgia

A systematic review of ACT in patients with fibromyalgia showed small-to-moderate effects in favour of ACT regarding pain, depression, anxiety, sleep and health-related quality of life (HRQoL) at the end of the treatment. The authors concluded that the health benefit effects were promising but uncertain.

A randomised controlled trial of 12 weekly ACT group sessions in patients with fibromyalgia showed the benefits in various domains at a 3-month follow-up; psychological flexibility was improved during treatment.

Another randomised trial comparing ACT with pharmacological treatment and waiting list showed that ACT was superior in patients with fibromyalgia and that the benefits were maintained at 6 months. However, the number needed to treat (NNT) for 50% improvement was 46 in this study, which was higher than expected for other treatments.

A cost-effectiveness trial of ACT in fibromyalgia using economic outcomes of HRQoL and healthcare use at 6-month follow-up showed that the ACT group had less direct costs than the pharmacological treatment group and waiting list group. The lower direct costs were due to fewer primary care visits and less medication costs.

A randomised trial of an 8-week ACT course compared with an education group was followed up for 12 weeks. Both groups showed differential patterns of success. The ACT group showed significant improvements in success in intimate relationships; both groups led to improvements in valued living. The authors concluded that different interventions might best suit certain valued domains.

Online ACT

A trial of online ACT showed a significant reduction in the impact of fibromyalgia. Improvements in pain acceptance mediated these. This study used an online ACT of seven modules over 8 weeks.

Guidelines

Recent NICE guidelines for chronic primary pain recommend that ACT be delivered by healthcare professionals who have undergone the appropriate training.

Key Points

- ACT enables a patient with fibromyalgia to accept and embrace the problem to improve the functional outcome.
- Relational frame theory: rational skills may not be effective when it affects psychology.
- Functional contextualism: looks at the whole event to improve functional outcome, aiding a more specific, meaningful clinical goal.
- Six core components of ACT: cognitive defusion, acceptance, being in the present moment, self as a context, values and committed action.
- Metaphors are commonly used in clinical practice in ACT.
- The evidence is variable, but NICE guidelines recommend ACT for chronic pain if delivered by a trained clinician.

References

1. Vasu T. Psychology in chronic pain. In: Vasu T, Balasubramanian S, Kodivalasa M, Ingle PM, Eds. *Chronic pain management*. Shrewsbury, UK: tfm publishing Ltd; 2021: pp. 183-7.

2. Twohig MP. Acceptance and commitment therapy. *Cogn Behav Pract* 2012; 19(4): 499-507.

3. Haugmark T, Hagen KB, Smedslund G, Zangi HA. Mindfulness- and acceptance-based interventions for patients with fibromyalgia – a systematic review and meta-analyses. *PLoS ONE* 2019; 14(9): e0221897.

4. Wicksell RK, Kemani M, Jensen K, *et al.* Acceptance and commitment therapy for fibromyalgia: a randomized controlled trial. *Eur J Pain* 2013; 17(4): 599-611.

5. Luciano JV, Guallar JA, Aguado J, *et al.* Effectiveness of group acceptance and commitment therapy for fibromyalgia: a 6-month randomized controlled trial (EFFIGACT study). *Pain* 2014; 155(4): 693-702.

6. Luciano JV, D'Amico F, Feliu-Soler A, *et al.* Cost-utility of group acceptance and commitment therapy for fibromyalgia versus recommended drugs: an economic analysis alongside a 6-month randomized controlled trial conducted in Spain (EFFIGACT study). *J Pain* 2017; 18(7): 868-80.

7. Steiner JL, Bogusch L, Bigatti SM. Values-based action in fibromyalgia: results from a randomized pilot of acceptance and commitment therapy. *Health Psychol Res* 2013; 1(3): e34.

8. Simister HD, Tkachuk GA, Shay BL, *et al.* Randomized controlled trial of online acceptance and commitment therapy for fibromyalgia. *J Pain* 2018; 19(7): 741-53.

9. National Institute for Health and Care Excellence; 2021. Chronic pain (primary and secondary) in over 16s: assessment of all chronic pain and management of chronic primary pain. NICE guideline, NG193. Available from: http://www.nice.org.uk/guidance/ng193/chapter/recommendations.

Fibromyalgia

Chapter 57

Mindfulness-based therapies

Introduction

Mindfulness-based psychological therapies are newer-generation talking therapies that focus on the present moment rather than dwelling on multiple problems and catastrophising. The attention is non-judgemental in mindfulness-based approaches.

Practicalities

Patients with fibromyalgia must be fully aware of where they are and what they are doing, rather than being overwhelmed by what is happening outside.

This could be achieved using meditation techniques, breathing strategies, and regular practice of mindfulness. The patient is facilitated to live in, and concentrate on, the present moment. This is done using any of the senses, including touch, sight, sound, taste, or smell. This approach creates awareness of thoughts in the present moment.

Components of mindfulness

Mindfulness consists of two components:

- Self-regulation of attention.
- Acceptance of one's own experiences in a non-evaluative way (non-reactive awareness).

In patients with fibromyalgia, mindfulness enables them to relate to the pain without suffering. It cultivates an attitude of kindness, acceptance, generosity and patience towards unpleasant emotions and thoughts.

Mindfulness-based stress reduction

Mindfulness-based stress reduction (MBSR) follows the ancient spiritual practice of mindfulness but is not tailored to any particular diagnosis. In patients with fibromyalgia, it focuses on intensive mindfulness meditation training and a discussion on stress and life skills.

Mindfulness-based cognitive therapy

Mindfulness-based cognitive therapy (MBCT) integrates MBSR with cognitive behavioural therapy (CBT). In contrast with MBSR, MBCT targets specific conditions and emphasises the psychological aspects of the experience.

Evidence for mindfulness-based therapies

A systematic review of mindfulness-based interventions, including MBSR and MBCT in patients with fibromyalgia, showed small-to-moderate effects in favour of these interventions regarding pain, depression, anxiety, sleep and health-related quality of life (HRQoL) at the end of the treatment. The authors concluded that the health benefit effects are promising but uncertain.

Another systematic review looked at six trials and found low-quality evidence for short-term improvement of quality of life with MBSR in patients with fibromyalgia. Therefore, the authors could only make a weak recommendation for MBSR in fibromyalgia.

A three-armed randomised trial in patients with fibromyalgia that compared MBSR in an active control group and in a waiting list group showed that MBSR did not improve the primary outcome of improving HRQoL. However, it showed a benefit in secondary outcomes of symptom relief.

An experimental trial using a mindfulness-based training programme in a waiting list control group of patients with fibromyalgia showed a statistically significant reduction in anger (trait) levels, internal expression of anger, state anxiety and depression compared with the control group. In addition, these results showed that the mindfulness-based treatment was effective after 7 weeks, and the benefits were maintained for 3 months after the end of the intervention.

A cost-utility analysis study of MBSR in patients with fibromyalgia compared with multicomponent therapy and usual care showed that MBSR achieved a significant reduction in costs compared with other study arms, especially in terms of indirect costs and primary healthcare services; this randomised study looked at costs over 12 months.

A 3-year follow-up analysis of MBSR participants with fibromyalgia showed sustained benefits in various measures, including pain scores, quality of life, coping levels, anxiety, depression and somatic complaints.

Guidelines

The European League Against Rheumatism (EULAR) gives a weak recommendation for mindfulness-based approaches. It quotes a meta-analysis of six reviews including 13 trials that showed that MBSR resulted in improvements in pain.

Key Points

- Mindfulness involves being fully aware of the present without being overwhelmed by what is happening outside.
- It involves two components: self-regulation of attention and accepting experiences without any judgement.
- MBSR involves the traditional spiritual meditation practice without tailoring this to a particular diagnosis.
- MBCT involves cognitive therapy along with mindfulness.
- The evidence for mindfulness in fibromyalgia is variable. EULAR gives a weak recommendation for mindfulness in fibromyalgia.

References

1. Vasu T. Psychology in chronic pain. In: Vasu T, Balasubramanian S, Kodivalasa M, Ingle PM, Eds. *Chronic pain management*. Shrewsbury, UK: tfm publishing Ltd; 2021: pp. 183-7.

2. Haugmark T, Hagen KB, Smedslund G, Zangi HA. Mindfulness- and acceptance-based interventions for patients with fibromyalgia – a systematic review and meta-analyses. *PLoS ONE* 2019; 14(9): e0221897.

3. Lauche R, Cramer H, Dobos G, *et al.* A systematic review and meta-analysis of mindfulness-based stress reduction for the fibromyalgia syndrome. *J Psychosom Res* 2013; 75(6): 500-10.

4. Schmidt S, Grossman P, Schwarzer B, *et al.* Treating fibromyalgia with mindfulness-based stress reduction: results from a 3-armed randomized controlled trial. *Pain* 2011; 152(2): 361-9.

5. Amutio A, Franco C, de Carmen Perez-Fuentes M, *et al.* Mindfulness training for reducing anger, anxiety, and depression in fibromyalgia patients. *Front Psychol* 2015; 5: 1572.

6. Pérez-Aranda A, D'Amico F, Feliu-Soler A, *et al.* Cost-utility of mindfulness-based stress reduction for fibromyalgia versus a multicomponent intervention and usual care: a 12-month randomized controlled trial (EUDAIMON study). *J Clin Med* 2019; 8(7): 1068.

7. Grossman P, Tiefenthaler-Gilmer U, Raysz A, Kesper U. Mindfulness training as an intervention for fibromyalgia: evidence of postintervention and 3-year follow-up benefits in well-being. *Psychother Psychosom* 2007; 76(4): 226-33.

8. Macfarlane GJ, Kronisch C, Dean LE, *et al.* EULAR revised recommendations for the management of fibromyalgia. *Ann Rheum Dis* 2017; 76(2): 318-28.

Chapter 58

Other psychological therapies

Introduction

Other psychological therapies, such as psychodynamic therapy, dialectical behaviour therapy, experiential therapy, meditation therapy, hypnotherapy, eye movement desensitisation and reprocessing (EMDR) therapy and exposure therapy, have been trialled in fibromyalgia, but the evidence is variable.

Meditation-based psychotherapy

International consensus guidelines on patients with fibromyalgia have recommended meditation-based psychotherapy as effective in improving depression symptoms following a 1-weekly session for 8 weeks. In addition, they recommended therapy for patients with complex emotional needs, especially in constructs such as catastrophising.

The European League Against Rheumatism (EULAR) guidelines looked at six reviews with eight trials focusing on qigong, yoga, tai chi, or a combination of these therapies. They found insufficient evidence to make individual recommendations. In conclusion, EULAR made a 'weak for' recommendation for meditation-based movement therapies.

Hypnotherapy

Hypnotherapy is a mind-body intervention that creates a state of focused attention and increased suggestibility in treating a disorder (see Chapter 38 for details).

The EULAR gave a weak recommendation against the use of hypnotherapy; it examined a review of four trials, and the results were variable.

Psychodynamic and psychoanalytic therapy

These interventions aim to change behaviours and feelings by finding the unconscious meaning or motivation of the exposure. Graded exposure helps to uncover and expose feelings.

A randomised trial of patients with fibromyalgia who also had comorbid depression or anxiety and used 25 sessions of psychodynamic therapy was compared with patients undergoing routine management. The study failed to show any marked superiority in psychodynamic therapy.

Compassion therapy

Compassion-focused therapy encourages patients with fibromyalgia to be compassionate and kind toward themselves and others. While CBT focuses on thinking and behaviour, compassion therapy focuses on the emotion behind these thoughts.

A randomised trial of compassion therapy versus relaxation therapy in fibromyalgia showed that attachment-based compassion therapy resulted in larger improvements in quality of life and was less costly after their 8-week treatment.

Eye movement desensitisation and reprocessing (EMDR)

EMDR is used in patients with fibromyalgia who also have post-traumatic stress disorder (PTSD). This approach helps to reprocess the traumatic memories to reduce their impact. It entails a risk of worsening the distress and needs to be approached by a qualified clinician.

A systematic review of EMDR in chronic pain patients concluded that there was insufficient evidence to recommend the treatment. There are isolated case reports of EMDR in fibromyalgia, but the available evidence is of low quality.

Human givens therapy

Just like the physical needs of human beings, such as food, water, air and sleep, there are innate emotional needs that are essential. The human givens theory proposes that an imbalance of emotional needs can lead to problems.

The human givens theory includes nine emotional needs: security, attention, sense of autonomy and control, being emotionally connected with others, being part of a wider community, intimacy (friendship, fun, love), a sense of status within a social group, a sense of competence and achievement, and meaning/purpose. It involves the role of sleep and dreams in maintaining this state.

The scientific evidence is limited for the human givens therapy for patients with fibromyalgia.

Key Points

- Various psychological therapies have been trialled, but the evidence is limited in fibromyalgia.
- The EULAR gives a weak recommendation for meditation-based psychotherapy and a weak recommendation against hypnotherapy.
- Compassion therapy focuses on being kind to yourself and others.
- There is insufficient evidence for EMDR and the human givens approaches, but these have been trialled in case reports in the published literature.

References

1. De Miquel CA, Campayo JG, Flórez MT, *et al.* Interdisciplinary consensus document for the treatment of fibromyalgia. *Actas Esp Psiquiatr* 2010; 38(2): 108-20.

2. Macfarlane GJ, Kronisch C, Dean LE, *et al.* EULAR revised recommendations for the management of fibromyalgia. *Ann Rheum Dis* 2017; 76(2): 318-28.

3. Scheidt CE, Waller E, Endorf K, *et al.* Is brief psychodynamic psychotherapy in primary fibromyalgia syndrome with concurrent depression an effective treatment? A randomized controlled trial. *Gen Hosp Psychiatry* 2013; 35(2): 160-7.

4. D'Amico F, Feliu-Soler A, Montero-Marín J, *et al.* Cost-utility of attachment-based compassion therapy (ABCT) for fibromyalgia compared to relaxation: a pilot randomized controlled trial. *J Clin Med* 2020; 9(3): 726.

5. Tesarz J, Leisner S, Gerhardt A, *et al.* Effects of eye movement desensitization and reprocessing (EMDR) treatment in chronic pain patients: a systematic review. *Pain Med* 2014; 15(2): 247-63.

6. Griffin J, Tyrell I. Appreciating our biological inheritance. In: Griffin J, Tyrell I, Eds. *Human givens: the new approach to emotional health and clear thinking*, 2nd ed. Chalvington: Human Givens Publishing Ltd; 2013: p. 97.

Chapter 59

Improving sleep in fibromyalgia

Introduction

Sleep problems are common in patients with fibromyalgia. Some theories, such as the human givens theory, have proposed that sleep problems could be one of the factors predisposing susceptible patients to fibromyalgia. However, these problems could also be the result of the disease or the side effects of treatments such as medications.

An internet survey of 2596 patients with fibromyalgia asked them to rank their symptom intensity; the patients ranked non-restorative sleep (6.8) as worse than pain (6.4) and other central nervous system symptoms.

Vicious cycle

Poor sleep can lead to more fatigue and pain, creating a vicious cycle leading to the persistence of fibromyalgia. Pain can prevent patients from getting enough rest or sleep; sleep deprivation can also exacerbate the tender points and lead to tiredness.

Pathophysiology of sleep problems

Sleep studies have shown that patients with fibromyalgia experience wakefulness during the non-rapid eye movement (NREM) stage, leading to fewer periods of slow-wave sleep.

Poor sleep has been shown to cause aberrant glial cell activation and a subsequent low-grade neuroinflammatory state, associated with elevated levels of brain-derived neurotrophic factor (BDNF), interleukin-1β (IL-1β) and tumour necrosis factor alpha (TNF-α). These pro-inflammatory markers can induce central sensitisation, which is the key pathogenetic factor in fibromyalgia.

The abnormal brain metabolism of serotonin has been proposed to cause sleep arousal. This is relieved by pharmacological agents such as selective serotonin reuptake inhibitors (SSRI) and tricyclic antidepressants.

Sleep deprivation impairs the descending inhibitory pain modulating pathways, and leads to poor control and coping strategies in patients with fibromyalgia.

Insomnia is associated with grey matter atrophy in the cerebral cortex seen in magnetic resonance imaging (MRI) scan studies in patients with fibromyalgia; these changes were reversible with treatment for fibromyalgia.

Polysomnography

Sleep-recording studies have shown reduced sleep efficiency and an increased number of awakenings in patients with fibromyalgia. Reduced amounts of slow-wave sleep and an abnormal alpha wave intrusion in NREM sleep are termed alpha-delta sleep.

Electroencephalography (EEG) studies have also shown a high frequency of arousals and increased alpha-K complex levels, which are indicators of fragmented sleep.

Alpha-EEG sleep anomalies are associated with non-restorative sleep, but this is non-specific for fibromyalgia, as these can also be seen in patients with stage 4 sleep deprivation due to other causes.

Patients with fibromyalgia can also experience sleep apnoea or periodic leg movements.

Non-restorative sleep and daytime fatigue

Non-restorative sleep is considered a key diagnostic feature in fibromyalgia; it is a subjective perception of poor sleep quality and the state of being unrefreshed upon awakening. A study documenting 21-day electronic sleep diaries in 220 patients with fibromyalgia showed that the previous night's non-restorative sleep and morning pain catastrophising were directly related to end-of-day activity interference; these two factors were risk factors for greater daily pain levels.

Sleep problems in fibromyalgia

A 1-year follow-up study of patients diagnosed with fibromyalgia showed that most patients (94–96%) had problems with sleep. This study highlighted the high prevalence of sleep problems and their role in exacerbating fibromyalgia symptoms. In addition, the authors concluded that patients' sleep problems might be related to depression through pain and physical functioning.

Sleep, pain and fatigue

A daily analysis of 50 women with fibromyalgia showed that their social-interpersonal goal pursuits were affected if pain and fatigue were worse on that day. Non-restorative sleep on the previous night predicted the progress towards health-fitness goals in these patients. Achieving social-interpersonal goals was linked to a positive mood in patients throughout the day.

Ways to improve sleep in fibromyalgia

Finding ways to reduce stress will improve sleep quality; the following measures can help, but the patient with fibromyalgia should be informed that these actions will take a few weeks before a change is seen:

- Set up a regular sleep schedule, including fixing the same time to go to bed and wake up every day, including weekends, to enable streamlining of circadian rhythms.

- Avoid using a mobile phone/laptop in the bedroom; avoid these devices for at least 1 hour before bed.
- Avoid watching television or listening to loud noise before going to bed.
- Set an appropriate temperature in the bedroom, not warm, but slightly colder.
- Avoid consuming caffeine or sparkling drinks for 2 hours before going to bed.
- Set aside time to wind down before bed, read relaxing books, listen to relaxing music, etc.
- Perform breathing exercises before bedtime.
- Sit in mindfulness meditation before bedtime.
- Have a comfortable mattress and bedding.
- Avoid daytime naps; if needed, restrict these to less than 30–60 minutes.
- Avoid alcohol in the evening.
- Restrict fluid intake for 1–2 hours before bed to reduce the need to wake up for the toilet.
- Taking a warm bath before bedtime can help.
- Exercise is good, but it is better done earlier in the day rather than in the evening.
- Blue light filters for mobile phones can reduce eye strain, improve sleep patterns and improve melatonin secretion.

Cognitive behavioural therapy (CBT) for insomnia (CBT-i)

Specific CBT therapy for insomnia (CBT-i) has been trialled under various conditions and is considered a first-line treatment for primary insomnia.

A randomised controlled trial of CBT-i in patients with fibromyalgia showed improvements in sleep quality, anxiety and depression compared with non-pharmacological treatments. Still, there was no improvement in sleep efficiency. However, another randomised trial comparing CBT-i with a sleep hygiene education programme showed that CBT-i had significant greater benefits. In contrast, an education group only reported improved sleep quality, whereas the CBT-i group improved in other domains including fatigue, daily functioning, pain catastrophising, anxiety and depression.

A study compared CBT-i with CBT for pain (CBT-p) and found that CBT-i was the better choice as improvements were larger and lasted longer. Another study using MRI compared both these interventions regarding cortical thickness changes in the brain; the CBT-i group showed a slowing or reversing of cortical grey matter atrophy in patients with fibromyalgia and insomnia.

Role of melatonin

Melatonin is secreted by the pineal gland, and its secretion increases in darkness in the evening or at nighttime; melatonin helps to regulate circadian rhythms. Melatonin facilitates a transition to sleep and promotes good quality sleep. Some studies have even proposed low melatonin levels to be one of the aetiological factors in fibromyalgia; but there is argument whether it is the cause or an associated factor.

A systematic review on the use of melatonin in patients with fibromyalgia reported positive effects but noted significant heterogeneity among the included studies.

A randomised trial of a 3mg dose of melatonin at bedtime in patients with fibromyalgia showed significant improvements in reducing tender points and pain severity and in improving sleep and global assessment. Another trial compared different doses of melatonin with or without fluoxetine and concluded that both doses of melatonin at 3 and 5mg/day in combination with 20mg/day of fluoxetine resulted in a significant reduction in Fibromyalgia Impact Questionnaire (FIQ) scores.

Role of vitamin D supplements

Vitamin D has both a direct and indirect role in sleep regulation; its receptors are expressed in areas of the brain that have a role in sleep regulation. Indirectly, it is involved in melatonin production pathways, which have a major role in circadian rhythm maintenance. A randomised study looked at patients with fibromyalgia who had low vitamin D levels; the correction by supplementing vitamin D was compared with a control group. Treatment with vitamin D produced a marked reduction in pain over the treatment period.

Role of sleep medications

An internet survey of patients with fibromyalgia showed that they used medications for sleep such as zolpidem (41%), alprazolam (33%), diazepam (28%) and clonazepam (25%), but they reported good efficacy at 64%, 70%, 65% and 61%, respectively. These quoted results were higher than for many other neuropathic and antidepressant medications. However, the scientific evidence for sleep medications in patients with fibromyalgia is limited.

These medications can be habit-forming and can have undesirable side effects. They can cause excessive daytime sleepiness and central nervous system effects. In addition, parasomnia is a disruptive sleep-related disorder that can occur with medications.

Key Points

- Sleep problems are common in fibromyalgia; non-restorative sleep is typical in fibromyalgia.
- Wakefulness during NREM sleep, less slow-wave sleep and alpha-EEG sleep abnormalities are common in fibromyalgia.
- Sleep improvement measures should be a definite part of the comprehensive management plan for fibromyalgia.
- CBT-i produced better results than CBT-p in fibromyalgia.
- Melatonin has a role in restoring circadian rhythms and sleep.

References

1. Bennett RM, Jones J, Turk DC, *et al.* An internet survey of 2,596 people with fibromyalgia. *BMC Musculoskelet Disord* 2007; 8: 27.

2. Nijs J, Loggia ML, Polli A, *et al.* Sleep disturbances and severe stress as glial activators: key targets for treating central sensitization in chronic pain patients? *Expert Opin Ther Targets* 2017; 21(8): 817-26.

3. Choy EHS. The role of sleep in pain and fibromyalgia. *Nat Rev Rheumatol* 2015; 11(9): 513-20.

4. Dauvilliers Y, Touchon J. Sleep in fibromyalgia: review of clinical and polysomnographic data. *Neurophysiol Clin* 2001; 31(1): 18-33.

5. McCrae CS, Mundt JM, Curtis AF, *et al.* Gray matter changes following cognitive behavioral therapy for patients with comorbid fibromyalgia and insomnia: a pilot study. *J Clin Sleep Med* 2018; 14(9): 1595-603.

6. Mun CJ, Davis MC, Campbell CM, *et al.* Linking nonrestorative sleep and activity interference through pain catastrophizing and pain severity: an intraday process model among individuals with fibromyalgia. *J Pain* 2020; 21(5-6): 546-56.

7. Bigatti SM, Hernandez AM, Cronan TA, Rand KL. Sleep disturbances in fibromyalgia syndrome: relationship to pain and depression. *Arthritis Rheum* 2008; 59(7): 961-7.

8. Affleck G, Tennen H, Urrows S, *et al.* Fibromyalgia and women's pursuit of personal goals: a daily process analysis. *Health Psychol* 1998; 17(1): 40-7.

9. Climent-Sanz C, Valenzuela-Pascual F, Martínez-Navarro O, *et al.* Cognitive behavioral therapy for insomnia (CBT-i) in patients with fibromyalgia: a systematic review and meta-analysis. *Disabil Rehabil* 2021; 14: 1-14.

10. Martínez MP, Miró E, Sánchez AI, *et al.* Cognitive-behavioral therapy for insomnia and sleep hygiene in fibromyalgia: a randomized controlled trial. *J Behav Med* 2014; 37(4): 683-97.

11. McCrae CS, Williams J, Roditi D, *et al.* Cognitive behavioral treatments for insomnia and pain in adults with comorbid chronic insomnia and fibromyalgia: clinical outcomes from the SPIN randomized controlled trial. *Sleep* 2019; 42(3): zsy234.

12. Hemati K, Amini Kadijani AA, Sayehmiri F, *et al.* Melatonin in the treatment of fibromyalgia symptoms: a systematic review. *Complement Ther Clin Pract* 2020; 38: 101072.

13. Citera G, Arias MA, Maldonado-Cocco JA, *et al.* The effect of melatonin in patients with fibromyalgia: a pilot study. *Clin Rheumatol* 2000; 19(1): 9-13.

14. Hussain SA, Al-Khalifa II, Jasim NA, Gorial FI. Adjuvant use of melatonin for treatment of fibromyalgia. *J Pineal Res* 2011; 50(3): 267-71.

15. Romano F, Muscogiuri G, Di Benedetto ED, *et al.* Vitamin D and sleep regulation: is there a role for vitamin D? *Curr Pharm Des* 2020; 26(21): 2492-6.

16. Wepner F, Scheuer R, Schuetz-Wieser B, *et al.* Effects of vitamin D on patients with fibromyalgia syndrome: a randomized placebo-controlled trial. *Pain* 2014; 155(2): 261-8.

Fibromyalgia

Chapter 60

Pain management programmes

Introduction

Pain management programmes (PMPs) are an integral part of the management strategies available in many pain services for patients with fibromyalgia. Most PMPs are based on cognitive behavioural principles and involve a group programme with multiple healthcare professionals. They promote physical, social, and emotional well-being; they aim to create a behaviour change to improve the quality of life (QoL) in patients with persistent pain due to fibromyalgia.

Objectives of a PMP

A PMP aims to provide skills and resources to patients for their self-management (ability to cope) of pain and to achieve as normal a life as possible in patients with persistent pain due to any cause by:

- Decreasing the emotional distress component in chronic pain.
- Reducing physical disability associated with chronic pain.
- Improving self-management.
- Decreasing their dependence on healthcare resources.

Structure of a PMP

A PMP involves multiple healthcare professionals, including pain physicians, physiotherapists, occupational therapists, specialist pain nurses and psychologists, with a mixture of shared and unique competencies. In addition, other specialists such as pharmacists and previous participant patients as guides can also be involved to enhance the impact of a PMP.

In a usual set-up, PMPs will include chronic pain patients of multiple diverse aetiologies, including mechanical spinal pain, widespread pain such as fibromyalgia, neuropathic pain, post-surgical persistent pain, pelvic pain and facial pain, and pain due to other causes. However, the overarching principles are the same in that these look at improving the QoL by giving control back to the patient through self-management strategies.

There are four important aspects of a PMP:

- Education: on general health and well-being, pain physiology and psychology with an important focus on pain self-management.
- Guided physical therapy: activity management with an exercise component that involves appropriate and realistic goal setting.
- Guided behavioural change: identify unhelpful beliefs, thinking and habits to change a patient's behaviour to control their disability.
- Integration of learned skills in daily life: practically integrating the other aspects in daily life.

A PMP is usually delivered in a group format with 8–12 participants. Usually, the more time involved and the more intense is the PMP, the more chances there are of improving success rates.

Standard set-up of a PMP

The British Pain Society (BPS) recommends approximately 12 half-day sessions (36 hours); in clinical practice, usually this is spread over a 6- to 10-week period with 1 day a week of participation.

Variations in a PMP

An intensive residential PMP (15–20 days) can be delivered for significantly disabled or distressed patients. A specialist PMP needs some operational flexibility to inculcate individual psychology- and physiotherapy-based interventions, either before, during or after a PMP is completed, to optimise the results. This flexibility is particularly important for patients with fibromyalgia, as their needs can differ with a very diverse clinical presentation. A targeted early PMP predominantly comprises physiotherapy- and psychology-based interventions that can be used as a cost-effective strategy in the early stages.

Evidence for PMPs

There is level 1 evidence of a PMP's effectiveness in people with persistent pain. In terms of improving the pain experience, mood, coping, activity levels and a negative outlook in chronic pain, cognitive PMPs offer a better efficacy than standard treatment or no treatment (level 1 evidence).

There is also some evidence that PMPs reduce the chances of patients presenting to the accident and emergency department or primary care with pain-related problems. In addition, the incidence of patients being re-referred to specialist pain services and further use of pain medications is reduced with PMPs.

A randomised trial of a 1-week multidisciplinary in-patient self-management programme for patients with fibromyalgia showed no effect on psychological distress, functional/symptomatic consequences and self-efficacy.

Another randomised trial of a 6-week self-management programme for patients with fibromyalgia using pool exercises and education showed significant improvements in QoL and functional consequences, including fatigue, depression, psychological well-being, anxiety and vitality. Still, there was no change in pain levels.

Outcomes

Outcomes from a PMP in a patient with fibromyalgia need to be evaluated. An improved quality of life (QoL) and a return to work are important goals. Many services use various QoL-related questionnaires for auditing and assessing their outcomes.

Controversies due to National Institute for Health and Care Excellence (NICE) guidelines

NICE guidelines NG193 on chronic pain do not recommend Pmps; NICE quotes that most of the evidence for people with chronic primary pain did not show any difference in QoL when a PMP was compared with the usual care or waiting list controls. Furthermore, there were no benefits in any other outcomes. The Committee agreed that, due to the evidence and uncertainty about cost-effectiveness, they could not make a recommendation. This outcome was shocking to pain clinicians as the previous guidelines strongly recommended Pmps for chronic pain.

The Faculty of Pain Medicine (FPM) of the Royal College of Anaesthetists, London, UK, immediately expressed concerns regarding these guidelines; the FPM cautioned that there is a risk of decommissioning PMPs, as NICE does not recommended them.

Challenges

There is currently a restriction on services accessing a PMP. For a PMP to be successful, there are many practicalities, including development of a multidisciplinary team and the system to maintain it. Communication between primary care, referrers and the commissioning bodies can be challenging.

Internet-based PMPs

Online and web-based technologies are used in PMP delivery but these need to be evaluated for their evidence base. For example, a trial of internet-based self-management programmes was compared with usual care and assessed at 6 months and 1 year; at 1 year, the intervention group improved four out of six health status measures and self-efficacy. However, no differences in health behaviours or healthcare utilisation were found.

Key Points

- PMPs are an integral part of comprehensive pain management services.
- Important aspects of a PMP include education, guided physical therapy, behavioural change and the integration of learned skills into daily life.
- Usually, this is carried out in a group of 8–12 patients, spread over 6–10 weeks.
- The evidence for PMPs in fibromyalgia is variable.
- NICE guidelines do not recommend PMPs for chronic primary pain.

References

1. Ingle PM. Pain management programmes. In: Vasu T, Balasubramanian S, Kodivalasa M, Ingle PM, Eds. *Chronic pain management*. Shrewsbury, UK: tfm publishing Ltd; 2021: pp. 189-92.

2. The British Pain Society; 2013. Guidelines for pain management programmes for adults. An evidence-based review prepared on behalf of the British Pain Society.

3. Wilkinson P, Whiteman R. Pain management programmes. *BJA Educ* 2017; 17(1): 10-5.

4. Hamnes B, Mowinckel P, Kjeken I, Hagen KB. Effects of a one week multidisciplinary inpatient self-management programme for patients with fibromyalgia: a randomised controlled trial. *BMC Musculoskelet Disord* 2012; 13: 189.

5. Cedraschi C, Desmeules J, Rapiti E, *et al*. Fibromyalgia: a randomised, controlled trial of a treatment programme based on self management. *Ann Rheum Dis* 2004; 63(3): 290-6.

6. National Institute for Health and Care Excellence; 2021. Chronic pain (primary and secondary) in over 16s: assessment of all chronic pain and management of chronic primary pain. NICE guideline, NG193. Available from: http://www.nice.org.uk/guidance/ng193/chapter/Recommendations.

7.   Faculty of Pain Medicine; 2021. FPM concerns regarding new NICE chronic pain guidelines. Available from: https://fpm.ac.uk/fpm-concerns-regarding-new-nice-chronic-pain-guidelines.

8.   Lorig KR, Ritter PL, Laurent DD, Plant K. The internet-based arthritis self-management program: a one-year randomized trial for patients with arthritis or fibromyalgia. *Arthritis Rheum* 2008; 59(7): 1009-17.

Section 10

Guidelines for fibromyalgia

Fibromyalgia

Chapter 61

National and international guidelines

Introduction

Various national and international guidelines exist to aid the treatment and management of fibromyalgia, but these differ significantly in their recommendations. A few standard and commonly used guidelines are discussed in this chapter.

European League Against Rheumatism (EULAR) guidelines

EULAR published initial guidelines in 2007 primarily based on expert opinion, which was revised in 2017 with some newly available evidence. A multidisciplinary group from 12 countries assessed the available evidence.

Based on meta-analyses, exercise was the only 'strong-for' recommendation in these guidelines.

Based on expert opinion, the following main stages were suggested:

1. Initially, patient education and focus on non-pharmacological approaches.

2. If there is no response, other treatments (weak for as per meta-analyses) should be tailored specifically to the needs of the individual. This approach may involve:

- Psychological therapies (for mood disorders, unhelpful coping strategies).
- Pharmacotherapy (for severe pain or sleep disturbance).
- Multimodal rehabilitation programmes (for severe disability).

EULAR guidelines for medications

EULAR gave the following recommendations for medications:

- Amitriptyline: weak for, at a low dose.
- Pregabalin: weak for.
- Gabapentin: research only.
- Duloxetine, milnacipran: weak for.
- Tramadol: weak for.
- NSAIDs: weak against.
- Capsaicin: weak against.
- SSRI: weak against.
- Cyclobenzaprine: weak for.
- Growth hormone: strong against.
- Monoamine oxidase inhibitors: weak against.
- Sodium oxybate: strong against.
- S-adenosyl methionine: weak against.

EULAR guidelines for non-pharmacological therapies

- Acupuncture: weak for.
- Exercise: strong for.
- Massage: weak against.
- Cognitive behavioural therapy (CBT): weak for.
- Mindfulness: weak for.
- Multicomponent therapy: weak for.
- Hydrotherapy: weak for.

- Meditative movement: weak for.
- Chiropractic: weak against.
- Hypnotherapy: weak against.
- Biofeedback: weak against.
- Guided imagery: strong against.
- Homoeopathy: strong against.

Canadian guidelines 2012

Canadian guidelines for the diagnosis and management of fibromyalgia syndrome (2012) reflected a paradigm shift in their diagnosis; the guidelines recognised that fibromyalgia symptoms fluctuate over time and are characterised by widespread chronic pain. The guidelines emphasised diagnosis in the primary care setting, and, in particular, without specialist confirmation and the need for unnecessary investigations. Some of the vital recommendations include:

- Self-management, using a multimodal approach is key.
- Goals regarding health status and quality of life should be re-evaluated regularly.
- Psychological evaluation and/or counselling may be helpful.
- CBT, even for a short time, is beneficial.
- A graduated exercise programme is essential.
- Strong opioid use is discouraged.

German guidelines 2012

German guidelines from the Association of the Scientific Medical Societies in Germany (Arbeitsgemeinschaft der Wissenschaftlichen Medizinischen Fachgesellschaften e.V. [AWMF]) were coordinated by the German Interdisciplinary Association of Pain Therapy:

- Amitriptyline is recommended.
- In comorbid depression or anxiety, duloxetine is recommended.
- Duloxetine and pregabalin can be used if there is no comorbid mental illness.
- Strong opioids are not recommended.

American Pain Society guidelines 2005

The American Pain Society guidelines (2005) recommend aerobic exercise, CBT, amitriptyline, and multicomponent treatment.

Key Points

- The initial guidelines of EULAR in 2007 were revised in 2017 after more important evidence was available.
- EULAR strongly recommends 'for' exercise in fibromyalgia.
- Self-management is key in most recent recommendations.

References

1. Macfarlane GJ, Kronisch C, Dean LE, et al. EULAR revised recommendations for the management of fibromyalgia. Ann Rheum Dis 2017; 76(2): 318-28.

2. Fitzcharles MA, Ste-Marie PA, Goldenberg DL, et al. 2012 Canadian guidelines for the diagnosis and management of fibromyalgia syndrome: executive summary. Pain Res Manag 2013; 18(3): 119-26.

3. Sommer C, Häuser W, Alten R, et al. Drug therapy of fibromyalgia syndrome: systematic review, meta-analysis and guideline. Schmerz 2012; 26(3): 297-310.

4. Häuser W, Thieme K, Turk DC. Guidelines on the management of fibromyalgia syndrome – a systematic review. Eur J Pain 2010; 14(1): 5-10.

Section 11

Patient awareness

Fibromyalgia

Chapter 62

Referral criteria to a pain clinic

Introduction

Chronic pain services see only the tip of the iceberg in cases of fibromyalgia, as the majority are managed in the community by general practitioners and other healthcare providers. Some cases undergo an investigative pathway via the rheumatology pathway. Patients are referred to a pain clinic when all other causes have been ruled out and still the pain is persistent.

Referral

Pain clinics work in a biopsychosocial model looking at management strategies rather than at cure or diagnosis. As a result, many patients with fibromyalgia go through the 'revolving door' phenomenon of seeing many specialists who recommend a variety of diagnoses and investigations. As we discussed in Chapter 2, fibromyalgia is part of the spectrum of functional pain syndromes, and patients can present with various multisystem symptoms.

Going through the traditional medical model can lead to the persistence of suffering due to multiple investigations and interventions in a patient with fibromyalgia. Therefore, it is prudent to rule out sinister causes, believe the patient, and create an appropriate rapport, ensuring that the patient understands that the clinician believes their suffering and engages in a biopsychosocial pathway. Pain clinics are best suited for this objective.

Criteria: diagnosis

It is difficult to engage a patient in this biopsychosocial model if the patient is still waiting for further diagnostic investigations or is still not satisfied with the investigative pathway. It is acceptable for patients to still undergo investigations, but they should understand that the pain clinic is looking at improving their quality of life in a multimodal pathway.

It would be appropriate for the referrer to finish their investigations before the referral is carried out so it is easier to engage patients in the management pathway.

All the red flags (clinical indicators of possible serious underlying medical conditions that need urgent attention) should be ruled out by the referring clinician before contacting the pain clinic.

Criteria: patient expectation

It is appropriate for a clinician to meet the patient's expectations when they come to their clinic; if a patient comes with unrealistic expectations from a service, this leads to frustration for both the patient and the clinician.

Patient information leaflets, information on websites, video podcasts of what to expect from the service, etc., can lead to a better informed patient. An informed, educated patient can engage better in treatment, and this will lead to better compliance with the intervention.

Criteria: willing to engage in a biopsychosocial model

A referrer should clearly explain the limitations of the pain service and explain that the patient should expect management via the biopsychosocial model. This approach differs from the traditional medical model as it focuses on the patient as a whole and on managing pain rather than finding a cure.

Criteria: quality of life

As discussed in Chapter 2, fibromyalgia affects approximately 2% of the population; most pain services do not have the capacity to see all these individuals with fibromyalgia. Therefore, primary care in the community manages the majority of patients with the available resources if they are coping well and engaging in the self-management pathway.

However, if there has been a significant impact on the patient's quality of life, these patients should be referred to a pain service for a multidisciplinary approach.

If first-line management therapies in the community have failed, they should be referred to a pain service.

Exclusion criteria

Patients with significant mental illness or a history of substance abuse should be referred to the appropriate specialty rather than to a pain service.

If a patient is not keen to participate in the biopsychosocial pathway, it is not appropriate to refer them to the pain service.

Misdiagnosis in referrals

A multicentre study looked at underdiagnoses and misdiagnoses of fibromyalgia with referrals to a rheumatology clinic; out of 427 referrals, 57 were misdiagnosed as other musculoskeletal disorders. The study concluded that, although fibromyalgia is a well-known clinical entity, differential diagnosis with spondyloarthropathies, connective tissue disorders and inflammatory arthritis can still be a challenge for rheumatologists and general practitioners.

A review of patients referred to a multidisciplinary fibromyalgia clinic found that more than 32% of 457 patients in the study used opioids, and over two-thirds were being administered strong opioids. The authors found that labelling patients with fibromyalgia and using opioids led to negative health and psychosocial status. Opioid use in these patients was associated with lower education, unemployment, disability payments, current unstable psychiatric disorders, a history of substance abuse and previous suicide attempts.

Key Points

- Most patients with fibromyalgia are managed in the community/primary care.
- All red flags and treatable causes should be ruled out before referral to a pain clinic.
- Patients should be willing to engage in the biopsychosocial model if they agree to be referred to a pain service.
- Patients with fibromyalgia should be referred to pain services if their first-line therapy has not worked or their quality of life is affected.

References

1. Di Franco M, Iannuccelli C, Bazzichi L, *et al*. Misdiagnosis in fibromyalgia: a multicentre study. *Clin Exp Rheumatol* 2011; 29(6); Suppl 69: S104-8.
2. Fitzcharles MA, Ste-Marie PA, Gamsa A, *et al*. Opioid use, misuse, and abuse in patients labelled as fibromyalgia. *Am J Med* 2011; 124(10): 955-60.

Chapter 63

Clinical documentation

Introduction

Good clinical documentation is central to good medical practice in any clinical condition, including fibromyalgia; it is one of the key requirements of Good Medical Practice (GMP), published by the General Medical Council. GMP clarifies that clinical documentation must be clear, accurate and legible. In addition, personal information should be kept secure and in line with data protection law requirements.

What should this include?

GMP states that clinical records should include:

- Relevant clinical findings.
- Decisions made and actions agreed.
- Information given to patients.
- Treatments prescribed and investigations.
- Who should make the record and when?

Clinical documentation and communication

Appropriate clinical documentation is essential for continuity of care through communication between team members and others involved in the care of the patient with fibromyalgia. In addition, proper documented clinical communication improves the quality of the care delivered.

Legal aspect

Clinical documentation is an important aid for medicolegal implications. Please refer to Chapter 64 for more details.

Audit and governance

Clinical documentation is vital for an audit of a service; without appropriate records, it is impossible to audit a clinical intervention's outcomes and efficacy.

Clinical documentation and funding

Appropriate clinical documentation helps in accurate coding for the consultations, interventions, investigations, and other procedures carried out; this aids the coding team in procuring the correct funding for the services delivered by the hospital or service.

Need for good documentation

Clinical documentation should be:

- Simple and clearly written.
- Legible and easy to read.
- An accurate and true meaning of what was discussed and carried out.
- Maintained professionally.

Access to health records

Individuals with fibromyalgia have the right to access their health records. The UK Government has committed that patients should have access to their health records within 21 days of making a request.

Under the Data Protection Act (DPA) 2018, patients have the right to request access to their medical records under a subject access request without a charge. This right includes consent for information to be released to a third party such as a solicitor or insurance company and includes both paper records and digital records.

Key Points

- Good clinical documentation is key to GMP.
- Documentation should be clear, legible and accurate.
- Patients with fibromyalgia have the right to request access to their medical records under a subject access request and without a charge.

References

1. General Medical Council. Good medical practice; Updated November 2020. Available from: https://www.gmc-uk.org/-/media/documents/good-medical-practice---english-20200128_pdf-51527435.pdf.
2. UK Government, UK GOV. Data protection. Available from: http://www.gov.uk/data-protection.

Fibromyalgia

Chapter 64

Medicolegal aspects

Introduction

Clinicians and patients should be aware of the medicolegal aspects of fibromyalgia and chronic widespread pain symptoms. These aspects might be related to work, benefits, previous injury or accident and recovery issues.

Working group on medicolegal aspects

Medicolegal problems related to fibromyalgia have been discussed for more than three decades. In June 1993, an international working group conference was held in Norway to review these problems. Unfortunately, problems exist in the evaluation and recommendation of patients with fibromyalgia.

Challenges in diagnosis

Although the American College of Rheumatology guidelines helped in the definition criteria for fibromyalgia, these are not commonly used in clinical practice. Furthermore, there is a debate on whether coming to a diagnosis helps or not in patients with fibromyalgia. A true biopsychosocial model distances itself from having a diagnosis as such but tries to rule out sinister treatable causes.

Subjectivity of symptoms

All fibromyalgia symptoms, including pain, fatigue and brain fog, are subjective and are difficult to quantify. Therefore, although there are clear-cut diagnostic criteria (please refer to Chapter 14), the diagnosis of fibromyalgia is vulnerable to misuse due to this subjectivity.

A study assessing the previous jurisprudential analysis of the Ontario Workplace Safety and Insurance Appeals Tribunal pointed out that medical opinions were provided by clinicians who had not treated the patient before the alleged accident or injury and that they appeared to have relied solely on the patient's reporting of their symptoms.

Aetiological conundrum

Various aetiological theories are described in Chapters 5–10, but there is no single identifiable cause or precipitating factor. This problem could lead to the allegation of a trigger for fibromyalgia; it is difficult to prove or disagree with the theory of causation, and clinicians can feel overwhelmed when exceeding the sphere of their expertise.

Significant contributing factor

The legal concept of a significant contributing factor can be applied in workplace injury-related claims; legal practice requests the use of common sense in reaching a decision, alleging that the absence of factors other than the incident is insufficient to establish causality. This aspect could be argued and debated based on individual circumstances.

Challenges in identifying a disability

Challenges in the effect of fibromyalgia and its impact on disability benefits are discussed in detail in Chapter 65. Clinicians can be out of their depth when asked to assess if the fibromyalgia symptoms are severe enough to lead to compensation for the disability; they must be honest in declaring their limitations regarding this.

Complaints due to frustration

Patients with fibromyalgia can become frustrated with differing and conflicting opinions from different clinicians; this can lead to dissatisfaction and anger directed against the pain services, as patients expect a fix after waiting for long periods through this journey. A clear patient information leaflet explaining what to expect from the pain service and what is practically possible to achieve can reduce this distress.

Furthermore, the pain clinic should comply strictly with the biopsychosocial model, even if the patient's expectations are different from this pathway. This restriction should be explained empathetically and honestly, including apologies for the trouble taken by the patient. Patients with other expectations should be offered to be sent back to the primary referrer, after explaining the reasons, so that these patients can be channelled back along the pathway appropriate to their wishes.

Medicolegal claims of iatrogenic opioid addiction

Complaints have been documented on the toxicity, addiction and side effects of opioids in patients with fibromyalgia; careful evaluation is vital before starting any pharmacological agent in fibromyalgia. Patients should be informed in detail and alternative therapies should be offered and documented. Any intervention's benefit-risk analysis should be discussed and documented in the clinical records.

Key Points

- Medicolegal issues can be related to work, benefits, previous injury and recovery.
- Challenges in diagnosis and subjectivity of symptoms can make these issues more complex.
- Challenges in identifying disability can lead to frustration for both the patient and the clinician.

References

1. Wolfe F, Aarflot T, Bruusgaard D, *et al.* Fibromyalgia and disability: report of the Moss international working group on medico-legal aspects of chronic widespread musculoskeletal pain complaints and fibromyalgia. *Scand J Rheumatol* 1995; 24(2): 112-8.

2. Fitzcharles MA, Ste-Marie PA, Mailis A, Shir Y. Adjudication of fibromyalgia syndrome: challenges in the medicolegal arena. *Pain Res Manag* 2014; 19(6): 287-92.

Chapter 65

Disability benefits and fibromyalgia

Introduction

A patient with fibromyalgia should be aware of their rights to receive the appropriate disability benefits; the clinician and their team should be able to guide them through this process. The process and the pathway vary between different countries.

Quantification of disability

As the symptoms of fibromyalgia are subjective and self-reported, it is difficult to quantify the disability effects. However, functional impairment has a significant relationship with pain, psychological factors, work status, helplessness, education and coping ability.

Work disability claims

Remaining in work is very important for patients with fibromyalgia as it gives them identity and self-esteem. Work disability in a patient with fibromyalgia is a social problem. The affected patient has functional limitations that restrict their ability; at the same time, employers should be considerate and provide individualised solutions to help recovery.

A qualitative study of women with fibromyalgia concluded that society's capacity to help them adjust to their work environment and tasks is important for keeping them within the workforce.

Assessment for claims

Whilst a patient says they are experiencing pain and the clinician must believe what the patient is saying as fibromyalgia is such a subjective condition, any assessment for disability and claims has an objective to prevent the possible misuse of the social security system. There is added pressure from various bodies, including patient support groups, media and self-help organisations, and this can affect symptom presentation. This pressure should not allow the assessor to be prejudiced against the condition or be overly suspicious.

United Kingdom

The National Health Service recognises the existence of fibromyalgia as a specific disease; patients can apply for benefits and living allowance. The recent Government has changed the benefits system to allow universal credit payments every month to help with living costs. These payments are based on health conditions, disability, income and housing costs.

United States system

In 2012, the Social Security Administration published a protocol for a patient with fibromyalgia to claim a medically determinable impairment. This requires evidence for the 12-month period before the date of the application. After establishing the impairment, the intensity and persistence of symptoms are evaluated. Residual functional capacity (RFC) is assessed to determine whether any previous relevant work or other work could be performed. However, the system also recognises that fibromyalgia symptoms can fluctuate. Patient groups have stated that claiming benefits in this system is difficult for patients with fibromyalgia.

Since 2015, fibromyalgia has the official US International Classification of Disease (ICD)-10-CM diagnostic code of M79.7 Fibromyalgia.

Other countries

The Australian Government introduced new impairment tables to restrict disability benefits; they clarified that a medical condition should be fully diagnosed, stabilised, and treated in order to qualify for benefits. Fibromyalgia is not on the list of recognised disabilities approved by the Department of Social Services (2014).

The Canadian system allows benefits through the Canadian Pension Plan or private insurance companies. However, the Canadian Rheumatology Association and the Canadian Pain Society expressed concerns regarding the number of patients receiving disability benefits and quoted that some of these used the fibromyalgia diagnosis inappropriately.

Key Points

- Patients with fibromyalgia should be aware of their rights to disability benefits.
- The capacity of society to help these patients to adapt to their work is vital.
- Functional capacity determines the ability to do work or change accordingly.
- The UK Government introduced a universal credit system to aid support for benefits.

References

1.   Goldenberg DL, Mossey CJ, Schmid CH. A model to assess severity and impact of fibromyalgia. *J Rheumatol* 1995; 22(12): 2313-8.

2.   Van Houdenhove B. Fibromyalgia: a challenge for modern medicine. *Clin Rheumatol* 2003; 22(1): 1-5.

3.   Liedberg GM, Henriksson CM. Factors of importance for work disability in women with fibromyalgia: an interview study. *Arthritis Rheum* 2002; 47(3): 266-74.

4.   Schweiger V, Del Balzo G, Raniero D, *et al.* Current trends in disability claims due to fibromyalgia syndrome. *Clin Exp Rheumatol* 2017; 35(3); Suppl 105: 119-26.

Chapter 66

Patient support groups and forums

Introduction

A patient support group is a group of people with shared experiences and concerns who provide emotional and moral support to one another. It is much needed for people with fibromyalgia. See Chapter 22 for more details on networking in fibromyalgia.

Functions of a patient support group

Support for a patient with fibromyalgia has many functions, which include:

- Educate patients with fibromyalgia.
- Educate families and friends of these patients.
- Share the illness experience that comes with the broad spectrum of symptoms in fibromyalgia.
- Provide moral support to patients with fibromyalgia.
- Arrange discussions and talks either face to face or online.
- Invite specialist speakers to talk and explain the condition.
- Create awareness of available treatments or interventions amongst its members.
- Raise public awareness of the condition and its impact on the patients, their families, and society.
- Organise fundraising activities to help these individuals.

- Lobby for support for clinical needs with managers and healthcare policymakers in their local area, region, and country.
- Lobby parliaments/governments and politicians to raise awareness among political policymakers.

Guilt feeling

Patients with fibromyalgia lose their identity and can have feelings of guilt regarding this; furthermore, it can cause frustration regarding the loss this has made on physical, emotional, and financial aspects for themselves and their family. Talking or communicating in groups to share their feelings might help ease this psychological burden.

Fibromyalgia Action UK (FMA UK)

Fibromyalgia Action UK's (www.fmauk.org) motto is 'Fighting for freedom from fibromyalgia'.

Fibromyalgia Association UK was established in 1992 and merged with Fibro Action UK in 2015 to form the Fibromyalgia Action UK (FMA UK).

FMA UK is a charity run by volunteers, most of whom have fibromyalgia. FMA UK aims to make people aware of the condition, support those who experience it, and lobby for more effective, available treatments. FMA UK runs a national helpline and a benefits helpline; it has an online support forum available 24 hours a day/7 days a week. The charity produces many complimentary information booklets and videos to create awareness of fibromyalgia. FMA UK claims to work with over 150 support groups and has a network of regional coordinators to aid this work.

FMA UK organises events on International Fibromyalgia Awareness Day on the 12th of May.

Fibromyalgia Friends Together

Fibromyalgia Friends Together (fibro.org.uk) supports people with fibromyalgia and their carers, family and friends. They have an active Facebook group and face-to-face group meetings in regions.

Fibromyalgia Research UK

Fibromyalgia Research UK (www.fibromyalgiaresearchuk.com) organises many patient group meetings all over the UK in multiple regions. It also provides information on various aspects of fibromyalgia through its website

National Fibromyalgia Association (NFA)

The National Fibromyalgia Association (NFA) is a non-profit organisation with the aim of improving the quality of life for people with fibromyalgia. It assists local support groups and provides patient information and education. It publishes a magazine called *Fibromyalgia AWARE*. It has proclaimed the 12th of May as 'Fibromyalgia Awareness Day' and campaigns for the condition. It also supports research into the condition.

National Fibromyalgia & Chronic Pain Association (NFMCPA)

The National Fibromyalgia & Chronic Pain Association (NFMCPA; https://www.facebook.com/NFMCPA) is an American association that supports patients with fibromyalgia. Since 1998, it has embraced the 12th of May as Fibromyalgia Awareness Day to create awareness of the condition. It has a Facebook page with more than 173,000 followers.

Living with Fibromyalgia

Living with Fibromyalgia (livingwithfibro.org) is a group that supports the community for fibromyalgia

Support Fibromyalgia

Support Fibromyalgia is an American patient-centred non-profit organisation that educates and inspires the fibromyalgia community.

Fibromyalgia Association Canada

Fibromyalgia Association Canada aims to bring together people with fibromyalgia across Canada; it also wants to strengthen their presence and influence the government decision-makers regarding their healthcare.

Fibromyalgia Australia

Fibromyalgia Australia aims to fast track the improvement of medical healthcare for Australians living with fibromyalgia.

Participatory medicine

In modern times, patients and health professionals are actively collaborating and encouraging one another as full partners in healthcare; this action is called participatory medicine. This collaboration can lead to improved health outcomes, greater satisfaction, and lower costs. In addition, shared decisions lead to better-engaged patients, better compliance, and better results.

Evidence for online support groups

Online support groups can empower patients who participate in these groups. A study interviewing the online support group attendees that included patients with fibromyalgia showed that patients were empowered by exchanging information, encountering moral support, finding recognition, sharing experiences, helping others, and through enjoyment. The patients felt better informed and confident in their relationship with their physician, their treatment, and the social environment. This change led to an improved acceptance of the disease and increased optimism, self-esteem, social well-being, and control.

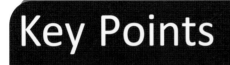

- Fibromyalgia patient support groups have patients who share similar experiences and provide emotional and moral support to each other in the group.
- They help to educate and create awareness about fibromyalgia.

References

1. Hu A. Reflections: the value of patient support groups. *Otolaryngol Head Neck Surg* 2017; 156(4): 587-8.

2. Society of Participatory Medicine. What is participatory medicine? Available from: https://participatorymedicine.org/what-is-participatory-medicine/.

3. Van Uden-Kraan CF, Drossaert CHC, Taal E, *et al.* Empowering processes and outcomes of participation in online support groups for patients with breast cancer, arthritis, or fibromyalgia. *Qual Health Res* 2008; 18(3): 405-17.

Fibromyalgia

Chapter 67

Questions and notes to make before visiting the pain clinic

Introduction

Information is key, and understanding the disease helps in recovery. Before a patient visits the pain service, it is essential that they are organised and prepared in order to get the maximum benefit from the consultation. This task can be overwhelming to plan after such a long wait and seeing so many specialists, but proper planning can help the patient take control of the situation.

Organising a fibromyalgia folder

Healthcare systems often do not communicate appropriately with each other, especially among different hospitals. The patient should take control of this situation, and it is prudent to organise a folder with all their earlier details. This folder can include letters/communication from a general practitioner and other specialists, records of investigations including blood tests and scans, a list of medications trialled, taken and their duration, effects of these medications and side effects, and a list of the chronological order of the disease and interventions.

Notes in preparation to the clinic

A patient with fibromyalgia might have seen many clinicians before visiting the pain service. Therefore, it is vital to prepare so that the patient has the correct expectations from the clinic and asks the right questions. Many pain clinics send an information leaflet on what to expect from the consultation; patients must read these leaflets a few times to understand the information and orient themselves.

Hospitals are vast and busy. It can be challenging to find the right place/clinic. Advise the patient to look at a map and be prepared for delays in car parking; it might be essential to reach the hospital at least 10–15 minutes in advance. Some pain clinics send questionnaires by post before the appointment or ask patients to fill these in while waiting in reception. These forms carry massive value for the clinician to understand the impact of pain on various domains.

Questions to ask in the clinic

Each patient will have different questions to ask the clinician. It is wise for patients to write a list of questions they want to ask in the consultation. A medical clinic consultation delivers vast amounts of information, and it can be challenging to remember everything. Most pain clinics send a copy of the clinical letter to the patient; if not, the patient has the right to ask for a copy of the letter to reiterate the information given in the clinic.

Patients can be nervous during the busy and challenging clinical consultation; writing down the questions that need to be asked helps in this situation.

Alternative treatments

A patient should clearly understand the side effects, limitations, and outcomes of an intervention. The clinician should provide and explain what alternatives are available, and if not, the patient should ask directly. Having been given a choice of treatments, the patient can choose treatment that matches their situation/convenience.

Key Points

- To maximise the benefit of a clinical consultation, a patient with fibromyalgia should prepare and organise themselves before this appointment.
- It is helpful for the patient to prepare a list of questions to ask, as the patient can forget questions during the busy consultation, especially if large amounts of new information are given.

References

1. Egeli NA, Crooks VA, Matheson D, *et al.* Patients' views: improving care for people with fibromyalgia. *J Clin Nurs* 2008; 17(11c): 362-9.

Fibromyalgia

Chapter 68

Patients — how to engage in pain services

Introduction

Patients must get the best out of their pain clinic appointment; to achieve this, a better understanding, good rapport with the clinician and better engagement can lead to better outcomes. Patient engagement is the action that individual patients must take to obtain the most significant benefit from the healthcare services available to them.

Engagement behaviours

The behaviours that help with engagement include information seeking, informed decision making, behaviours on navigating care, behaviours related to access to care (choosing the service), and maintaining personal health records.

Patients' expectation

Studies in patients with fibromyalgia have looked at the written responses to open-ended questions about their interactions with clinicians; most patients reported having positive interactions with their physicians. Suggestions for improving care included increasing supportive care, empathetic listening, and increased knowledge of alternative treatments.

Patients should research the difference between the traditional medical and biopsychosocial models used in the pain clinic. Reading the information leaflet from the pain clinic and doing some research can help in better engagement, as their expectations will match what can be delivered in the pain clinic.

Diagnostic delays

Studies surveying 800 patients with fibromyalgia and 1600 physicians across eight countries found that patients waited an average of 2.3 years before receiving their diagnosis of fibromyalgia; on average, they saw 3.7 different physicians before receiving their diagnosis. Most delays could be avoided by proper communication about their symptoms to the physician.

Openness

Clinicians should give alternative treatment options to a patient with fibromyalgia; treatment should be multimodal including, but not limited to, physical therapy, complementary therapies, medications, psychology-based approaches, group pain management programmes, injection therapies, occupational therapies, and others. Patients should be open and honest in clarifying their expectations and take their time before agreeing to a listing for a particular treatment. They have the right to take the time to discuss options with their family/friends or go back to their primary care clinician (general practitioner), who would know more about their long-term care before then agreeing to a treatment.

Health literacy

Patient information leaflets will help increase patients' engagement in the fibromyalgia service and improve their compliance with therapies. In addition, reading, understanding, and acting on these health information leaflets will help in better outcomes.

Shared decision making

Decision making regarding the management of fibromyalgia should never be unilateral or decided just by the clinician or the patient; this should always be done together. It is essential to include other stakeholders, including family/friends, the workplace, and other clinicians. Shared decision making involves patients and clinicians working together to select the appropriate therapy for that patient at that particular time.

Barriers to patient engagement

Time constraints in a busy clinic are a barrier to appropriate patient engagement; a patient with fibromyalgia should plan their pain clinic or any specialist clinic appointment appropriately (please refer to Chapter 67). Making notes and writing down questions a patient wants to ask before the clinic will help in this goal.

Key Points

- Patient engagement leads to the most significant benefit that can be achieved from available healthcare resources.
- Patients with fibromyalgia will be satisfied if their expectations match with what the healthcare service can deliver.
- Improving health literacy and shared decision making can improve outcomes in fibromyalgia.

References

1.   Gruman J, Rovner MH, French ME, *et al*. From patient education to patient engagement: implications for the field of patient education. *Patient Educ Couns* 2010; 78(3): 350-6.

2.   Egeli NA, Crooks VA, Matheson D, *et al*. Patients' views: improving care for people with fibromyalgia. *J Clin Nurs* 2008; 17(11c): 362-9.

3.   Choy E, Perrot S, Leon T, *et al*. A patient survey of the impact of fibromyalgia and the journey to diagnosis. *BMC Health Serv Res* 2010; 10: 102.

4.   Coulter A. Patient engagement – what works? *J Ambul Care Manage* 2012; 35(2): 80-9.

Chapter 69

Patients — how to form networks

Introduction

The clinician must guide patients to form their network or support groups in fibromyalgia. Most commonly, this opportunity should be used after attending group programmes such as pain management; this will empower the patient and help them take control of their pain and work together with their peers. Some of these networks also welcome friends and families to help understand and support their loved ones with fibromyalgia.

Studies have shown that influential patient participation groups and excellent service go hand in hand.

Patients taking control into their own hands

The goal of the management plan in the fibromyalgia service is to help the patient take control of their pain management into their own hands. Self-management should be assisted in a multimodal biopsychosocial pathway. Patient networks with the help of volunteers who have gone through this pathway can help guide other patients who have recently visited the pain service. This approach helps in better engagement of the patient in various interventions, as they will have a chance to discuss members of similar groups who have had similar experiences.

Local needs

Each patient participation group or network differs depending on local needs, availability, and resources. However, the goal is the same in sharing their experiences and supporting others through the same pathway in fibromyalgia.

How to set up a network

The most effective way to run a patient participation group or network is to have a core group of motivated patients who can establish and facilitate the group. Given the varying symptoms of fatigue, pain and distress in fibromyalgia, it can be challenging to run a patient network without a few core team members. The clinician should guide these individuals to provide the essential resources needed to run this network; giving space in the hospital or community can be an excellent start to run these groups face to face at regular intervals.

Characteristics of a good patient network

A good patient support network could include:

- Inclusive membership.
- Be representative of the disease population.
- Mutual understanding.
- A core committee with clearly defined roles.
- Supportive culture.
- A good relationship between the organisers.
- A clear pathway for accepting new patients.

A successful pathway can include the clinician staying away from the group but being there for support in case of need; the core committee will feel supported by this link between the network and the clinician. It can also be rewarding for the clinician and improve the relationship with their patients.

Key Points

- An effective fibromyalgia service should have a patient participation network or group.
- This approach helps patients to manage their pain themselves in a better way.

References

1. Medical protection. How to set up a patient participation group?; 2013. Available from: https://www.medicalprotection.org/uk/articles/how-to-set-up-a-patient-participation-group.

Fibromyalgia

Chapter 70

Workplace engagement

Introduction

Fibromyalgia is significantly associated with reports of working disability. For example, a case-control study showed that significant numbers of patients with fibromyalgia (46.8%) reported that they lost their job due to the disease, compared with only 14.1% of controls from non-rheumatology outpatient clinics.

Epidemiological studies have shown that nearly one-third (30.8%) of patients with fibromyalgia have a disability. Patients with disabilities were more likely to have been employed in manual professions or the service industry. In contrast, the remaining patients were more commonly working in non-manual jobs such as clerical/managerial or professional work.

Economic consequences

A United States study in 2005 compared the healthcare resources among employees with fibromyalgia with those of controls; total costs for employees with fibromyalgia (US$10,199) were significantly higher than for the controls (US$5,274). Fibromyalgia imposes a significant economic burden, and the authors concluded that the work loss contributed substantially to this effect. In addition, employees with fibromyalgia had more claims for psychiatric diagnoses, chronic fatigue, and most pain conditions.

Flag systems

Flag systems have been used in musculoskeletal conditions primarily, but the principles apply in fibromyalgia as this condition has similar features. Flags are a framework to identify factors that may become an obstacle in a patient's recovery and return to work. Early identification and attention to overcoming these can minimise the risk of work-related disability.

Red flags look at sinister or treatable causes. Orange flags look at mental health and personality disorders. Yellow flags look at psychological factors including perceptions, beliefs, and behaviours that could lead to chronicity. Black flags look at compensation or system factors, including disputes, financial strains, and the need to prove claim validity. Blue flags deal with work or social factors that are detailed below.

Blue flags

Blue flags can be due to work factors or social factors, such as:

- The perception that line managers or co-workers are not supportive of the rehabilitation process.
- Inflexible work needs, including not having the possibility to reduce work capacity.
- Low social support (low support from family, friends, or other networks).
- The social factor of poor communication, for example, a non-English-speaking patient in a Western country.

Managing work-related issues

Referral to an occupational therapist or workplace rehabilitation provider early in the recovery plan is vital. Patients should be informed and reassured;

active listening to acknowledge their concerns is essential. A clinician can challenge unhelpful beliefs, including catastrophising. A psychosocial assessment is vital early to assess the risk of poorer outcomes.

It is critical to communicate openly about the expectations for recovery and work. The occupational health specialist will contact the employer to understand their ability to accommodate a reduced work capacity or an altered work schedule or plan. A case conference between the patient, occupational therapist, and the employer can help in this openness.

Engagement with the workplace

Patients with fibromyalgia feel that suitable work should be paced so that they can perform their job well and with satisfaction, while keeping energy for home and free time and receiving acknowledgement and help from management and colleagues. Employers should be proactive in finding the employee's needs and discussing possible changes needed to adapt to the requirements of these patients.

Key Points

- Fibromyalgia is associated with disability and work-related issues.
- The incidence of disability is high for those with previous manual jobs.
- Blue flags relate to work and social factors that delay recovery.
- Engaging early in the workplace can help towards better recovery for the patient.

References

1. Al-Allaf AW. Work disability and health system utilization in patients with fibromyalgia syndrome. *J Clin Rheumatol* 2007; 13(4): 199-201.

2. Fitzcharles MA, Ste-Marie PA, Rampakakis E, *et al*. Disability in fibromyalgia associates with symptom severity and occupation characteristics. *J Rheumatol* 2016; 43(5): 931-6.

3. White LA, Birnbaum HG, Kaltenboeck A, *et al*. Employees with fibromyalgia: medical comorbidity, healthcare costs, and work loss. *J Occup Environ Med* 2008; 50(1): 13-24.

4. Western Australia workers' compensation scheme Government Agency. Using the flags model: a practical guide for GPs. Available from: https://www.workcover.wa.gov.au/wp-content/uploads/sites/2/2015/07/UsingTheFlagsModel_A_PracticalGuideForGPs_FinalAcess.pdf.

5. Bossema ER, Kool MB, Cornet D, *et al*. Characteristics of suitable work from the perspective of patients with fibromyalgia. *Rheumatology (Oxford)* 2012; 51(2): 311-8.

Section 12

Fibromyalgia in children

Fibromyalgia

Chapter 71

Fibromyalgia in children

Introduction

Unfortunately, the services available to help children with fibromyalgia are very sparse, even in developed countries. Educating healthcare professionals involved with children and adolescents regarding fibromyalgia is more complex, given that the biopsychosocial model is difficult to accept by many clinicians and parents of the child. More resources and facilities need to be established in a biopsychosocial model.

Why is it important to recognise and treat?

Fibromyalgia in children can have a disastrous impact on their quality of life, development, emotional and mental development, and learning skills and can impact their family significantly. However, if recognised and managed in a biopsychosocial pathway, integrating them back into their school life has a good prognosis.

Prevalence of fibromyalgia in children

Chronic pain is often found during epidemiological studies in children and results in high healthcare costs. A quantitative observational study looking at referrals to a paediatric chronic pain clinic (pain that lasted more than 1 year) showed that 14% of these patients had an initial primary diagnosis of fibromyalgia. This study showed that these children experienced a significantly worse health-related quality of life.

It has been published that 25% of new patients presenting to paediatric rheumatology clinics have idiopathic musculoskeletal pain, including pain due to juvenile primary fibromyalgia syndrome, which is often accompanied by markedly adverse functional and psychosocial impacts. In recent literature, the prevalence of musculoskeletal pain is reported as 32–40%, with an overall increasing prevalence or recognition of fibromyalgia in children.

The incidence of fibromyalgia in children is estimated at 4–6% of the population; an incidence of 6.2% was quoted in children aged 9–15 years. Another publication quoted the incidence as 5% in school-age children.

Prognosis in children

The outcome of fibromyalgia has been documented to be more favourable in children than adults; children tend to 'outgrow' the condition. Integrating the child back into their school environment to help continue their mental and social development will assist in achieving this goal of recovery.

Key Points

- The prevalence of fibromyalgia is approximately 4–6%.
- Children with fibromyalgia have a better prognosis compared with adults.
- It is essential to integrate children back into school life to help with their development and recovery.

References

1. Vetter TR. A clinical profile of a cohort of patients referred to an anaesthesiology-based paediatric chronic pain medicine program. *Anesth Analg* 2008; 106(3): 786-94.

2. Vetter TR. The epidemiology of pediatric chronic pain. In: McClain BC, Suresh S, Eds. *Handbook of pediatric chronic pain*. Springer Publishers; 2011: pp. 1-14.

3. Rusy LM. Clinical management of musculoskeletal pain syndromes. In: McClain BC, Suresh S, Eds. *Handbook of pediatric chronic pain*. Springer Publishers; 2011: pp. 96-9.

4. Zeltzer LK, Zeltzer PM. Chronic pain conditions. In: Zeltzer LK, Zeltzer PM, Eds. *Pain in children & young adults – the journey back to normal*. CA: Shilysca Press; 2016: pp. 54-6.

Fibromyalgia

Chapter 72

School engagement

Introduction

As mentioned in Chapter 71, integrating the child back into their school life helps in their mental and social development and aids in recovery from fibromyalgia. A school environment is essential for a child for optimal social development. Once a child is removed from the typical school routine, reintegrating them back into the school will be difficult and stressful.

School absenteeism

A prospective epidemiological study showed that school absenteeism was noted in 95% of children referred to a paediatric pain clinic; this caused significant functional disability. Furthermore, more than 50% of children had missed 5 or more days of school due to pain; most children attended school regularly after treatment in a multidisciplinary paediatric pain clinic.

Returning to school

There are challenges for a child or adolescent returning to school after an illness due to fibromyalgia. Some children require reasonable accommodation (environment, curriculum, equipment, and their functional limitations) to optimise functioning and decrease the likelihood of chronic boom and bust cycles. Children with fibromyalgia should be able to communicate efficiently to inform the need for a break from class.

Some children will need a part timetable to have flexible sessions that could help them integrate slowly into the regular routine. This step should be planned well according to the functional capacity of the child.

Individualised gradual return timetable

A proper multidisciplinary paediatric chronic pain team will have expertise from a specialist nurse who can liaise with school nurses or teachers to create a specific educational plan and help them gradually integrate into the routine. In addition, the child should have a specifically named advocate in the school to monitor and guide them in this pathway.

There should be contingency management in this time-bound gradual return plan. Any recovery plan can have relapses, common in a child with fibromyalgia with post-exertional fatigue that can worsen the pain. The expectations from the child should be reasonable and predictable; they should be mutually agreed upon by the child, clinician, parents, and the school authorities. The caregivers should make a promise to implement contingency plans if needed.

Recommendations for accommodations

When a child returns to school after a gap, they will need multiple accommodations that include:

- Medical accommodations: school teachers and friends should be able to understand their condition but at the same time avoid reinforcing medical thoughts; adherence to medications during school times; appropriate hydration, diet and unrestricted access to restrooms; an escape card that can be shown to teachers without any explanation if they want to go for a break to prevent a flare-up of pain.
- Physical accommodations: pacing strategies, scheduled breaks, carrying light weights, and assistive devices for learning. Some affected children might want to have a respite from physical education classes. Still, their presence in a different role could integrate them, to help teamwork but avoid strenuous games or activities.

- Psychological accommodations: a child with fibromyalgia needs validation of their distress; they should not be questioned to justify the extent of their pain. School counselling can help with comorbid anxiety and depression if needed.
- Academic accommodations: being off school for some time causes anxiety about catching up with the missed work; further ongoing work needs to be done, and it is easy for a child to become stressed and lose interest. A supportive educational plan should consider this so that it accommodates their needs.

Educating school staff

The teachers and school staff must be instructed that all pain is real. It is crucial to distract the affected child with fibromyalgia rather than asking if they are in distress; drawing more attention can enhance pain signals, and it is wise to distract in an empathetic manner. Any improvement is measured by increased functioning in day-to-day evaluation. It could be advised to focus on independence but continue using support when the child struggles. The staff should understand that a long-term problem needs a long-term solution.

Key Points

- Integrating a child with fibromyalgia into their school environment helps their social and mental development.
- A gradual return timetable to avoid flare-ups is essential when a child returns to school.
- Accommodations should be considered in medical, physical, psychological, and academic domains.
- Liaison between the clinical teams, the child, the parents and the school staff is vital to creating a workable plan that is reasonable and practicable; contingencies need to be planned if any relapse occurs in the recovery pathway.

References

1.   Vasu T. Leicester paediatric chronic pain service. *Pain News* 2016; 14(1): 35-7.

2.   Chalkiadis GA. Management of chronic pain in children. *Med J Aust* 2001; 175(9): 476-9.

3.   Oddo LE, Gray LS. Preparing for return to in-person school instruction in pediatric chronic pain populations. *Pediatr Pain Lett* 2021; 23(2): 17-23.

4.   Benore E, Fahernkamp A, Zhakunets O, *et al.* School re-entry following chronic pain and disability: a pathway to success. *Pediatr Pain Lett* 2020; 22(1): 2-15.

Chapter 73

Role of multidisciplinary paediatric pain clinics

Introduction

Multidisciplinary paediatric pain clinics help with a biopsychosocial model to aid a child with fibromyalgia in their recovery pathway. They consist of clinicians from various disciplines, as described in this chapter, with a single goal of helping the child recover.

Pain consultant

A pain consultant or anaesthetist with extensive experience in chronic pain in children usually leads the team. An initial multidisciplinary consultation usually takes 90 minutes or more, depending on the constituents of the clinic and their practicalities. A pain consultant is pivotal in educating the child and their parents in the biopsychosocial model and engaging in the treatment plan. In addition, the pain consultant takes responsibility for assuring the child and parents that the referring team have completed all diagnostic pathways and the need to engage in management rather than cure or diagnosis for further recovery.

The pain consultant usually uses a variety of metaphors to educate the child and the parents regarding the pathophysiology of chronic pain in fibromyalgia; this will create a better rapport, and better understanding and help in compliance with the treatment plans.

Specialist paediatric nurse

A paediatric nurse becomes the advocate for the child and takes the responsibility of conveying the child's thoughts and those of the family to the multidisciplinary team. The nurse also becomes the liaison for engaging the school nurse, teacher, school counsellor, or the school authorities and helps make adapted educational plans. Usually, the nurse also runs the drug review clinics, acupuncture clinics, and TENS machine clinics and takes an integral part in the pain management group programme for children. For example, in Leicester, UK, the team innovated with a distraction and relaxation programme for children aged less than 12 years that received a national award for excellence; the paediatric nurse and physiotherapist play an essential role in this workshop.

Paediatric physiotherapist

A specialist physiotherapist can engage the child in gradual mobilisation and remove the fear of movement. The child should be told that 'hurt does not mean harm' and the importance of desensitisation strategies should be stressed. The physiotherapist usually teaches breathing exercises to help with pain flare-ups, and the child is advised to practise these exercises regularly. The physiotherapist is also a vital part of the pain management group and the relaxation workshop. They also play a crucial role in examining the musculoskeletal system to assure the child and parents before engaging in the management pathway.

Paediatric psychologist

A psychologist is a critical part of the chronic pain team; in the initial appointment, they should assess the child's emotional needs. They are vital to evaluating safeguarding issues and determining the need for referral to a mental health crisis team. They play an essential role in informing the link between stress and pain in fibromyalgia, engaging children in the psychological pathway, aiding them in looking at the experience rather than pain, and directing them to self-management coping and counselling websites/apps. They should engage children in cognitive behavioural therapy

(CBT), acceptance and commitment therapy (ACT) or a mindfulness pathway and select appropriate patients for the group pain management programme.

Other clinicians

Depending on the funding and the resources available, the team will vary in structure. Other familiar healthcare professionals include paediatric consultants, paediatric rheumatologists, paediatric occupational therapists, social workers, play therapists and other staff.

Administrative staff

Any multidisciplinary paediatric pain clinic needs appropriate administrative staff to support the clinicians and be a link to the child and their parents. Parents are usually stressed and frustrated as the pain affects their child and the whole family. An empathetic administrative team can improve the satisfaction of the child and family. The staff also play an essential role in sending appropriate pain clinic leaflets before the consultation to advise the family on what to expect from the clinic; they should also send relevant questionnaires and triage forms to put in place a baseline assessment of psychological status.

Key Points

- A biopsychosocial model-based paediatric pain clinic needs multidisciplinary clinical staff with varied expertise.
- The structure of the team differs depending on the availability of knowledge and resources.

References

1. Vasu T. Leicester paediatric chronic pain service. *Pain News* 2016; 14(1): 35-7.

2. Faculty of Pain Medicine, Royal College of Anaesthetists. Relaxation and distraction workshop for 7-12-year old children in chronic pain and their parents. Available from: https://fpm.ac.uk/sites/fpm/files/documents/2019-07/Relaxation%20and%20Distraction%20Workshop.pdf.

Index